Heroes of the PANDEMIC!

~

Coloring Book

RIK FEENEY

This book belongs to:

____

Heroes of the PANDEMIC! Coloring Book

~ Rik Feeney

ISBN: 978-1-935683-27-8 (Paperback)

Richardson Publishing, Inc.
PO Box 162115
Altamonte Springs, FL 32716
www.RickFeeney.com
usabookcoach@gmail.com

Disclaimer:
Use this book assuming all risk for physical, mental, and social injury. The author and publisher accept no responsibility if you accidentally poke an eye out while coloring, suffer physical illness from ingesting crayons or sucking on felt tip pens, or lose sleep due to horrific nightmares of the pandemic. Please note the author and publisher spend every day running a metal detector up and down the beach in search of treasure. So far – zip, so suing either one of us may get you a barely functioning metal detector, two Speedo's and boxer shorts with torn elastic. Bottom line: We don't have squat, so you ain't going to get squat.

Permissions:
Vecteezy.com Pro License

Dedication:

This book is dedicated to: "All the Heroes" that have worked tirelessly to help their fellow man and woman and to the future where "Normal" looks something like what we were used to experiencing.

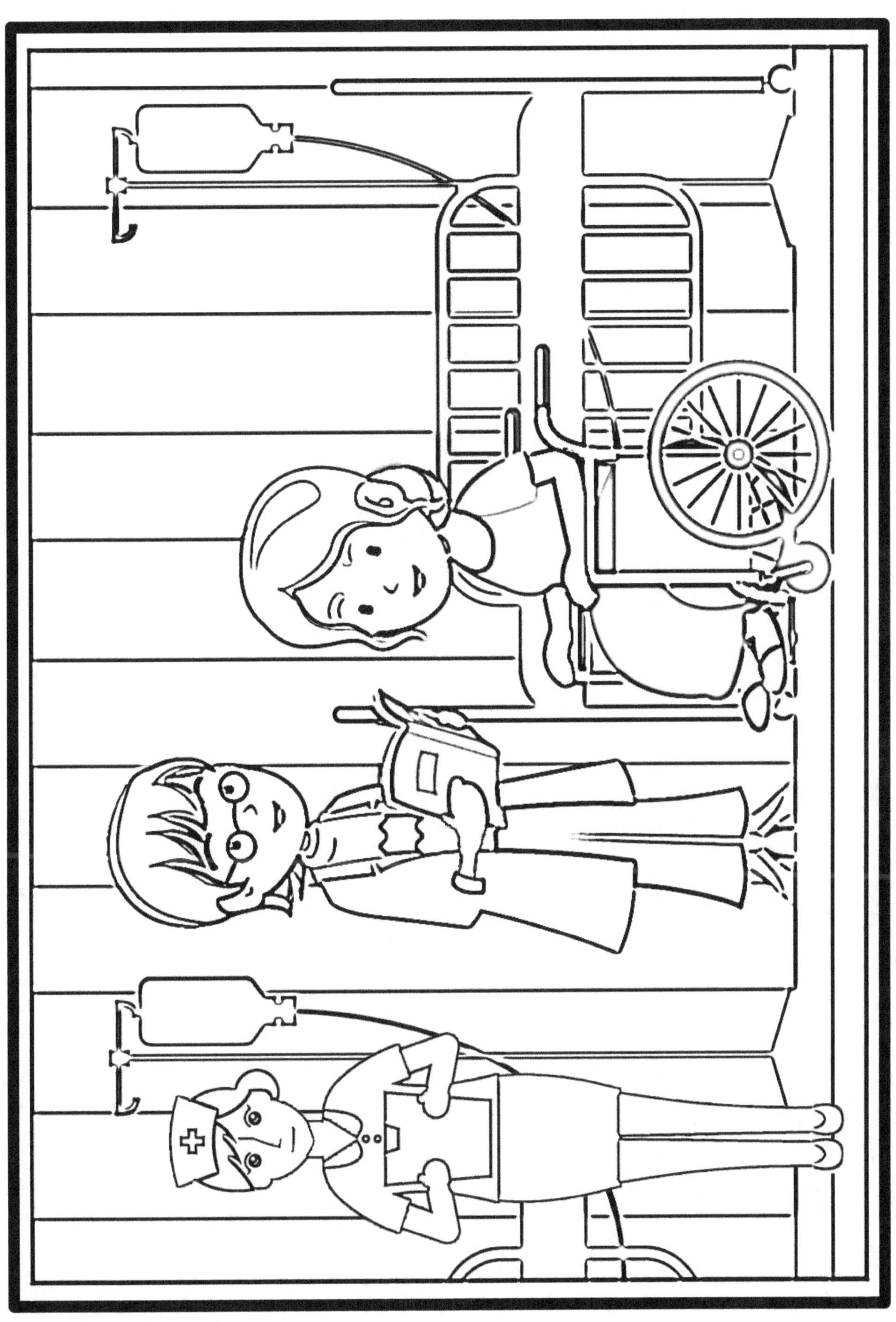

Artist Name: _______________

Date: _______________

Title: _______________

Dedicated to: _______________

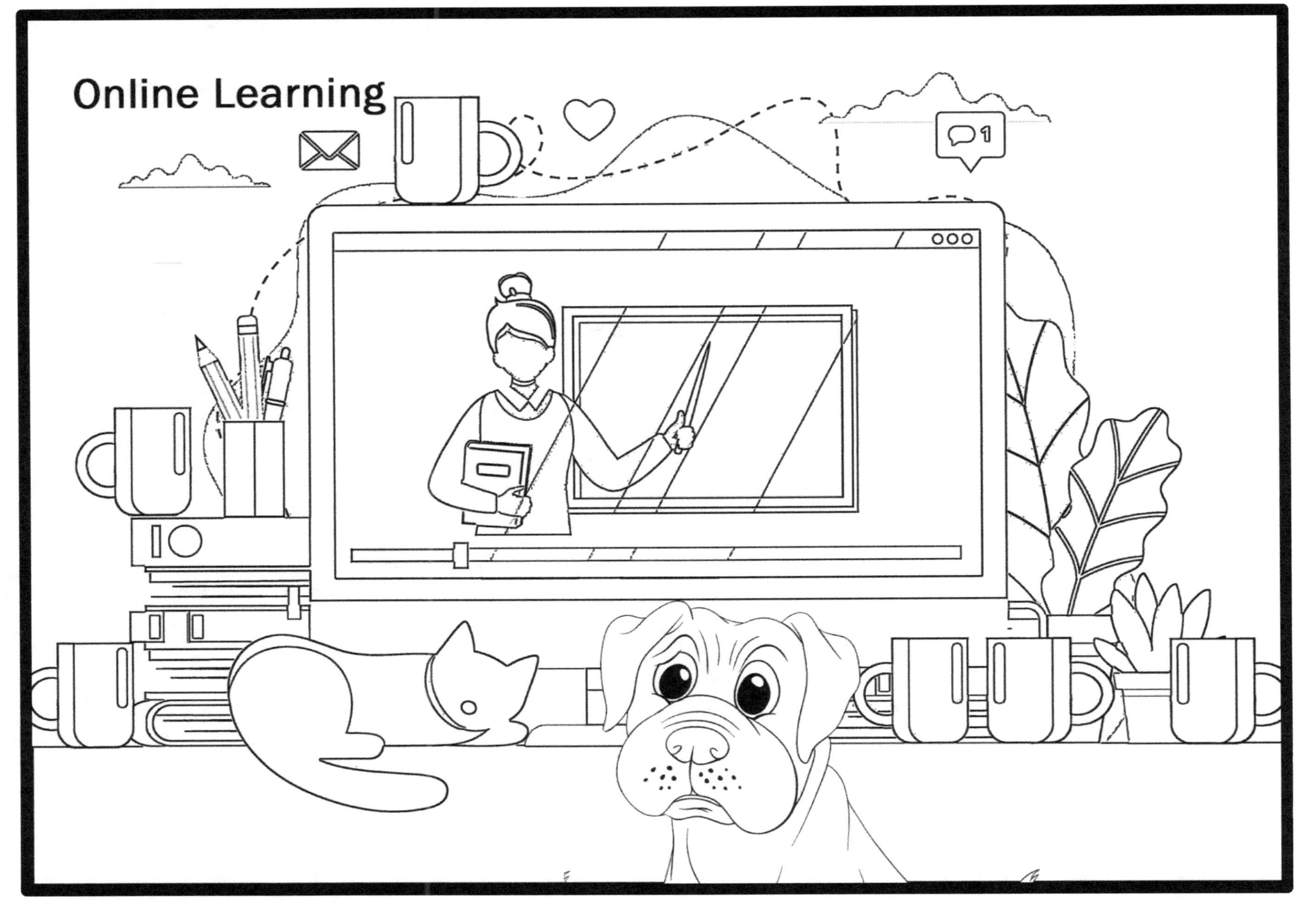
Online Learning

Artist Name:______________________

Date:______________________

Title:______________________

Dedicated to:______________________

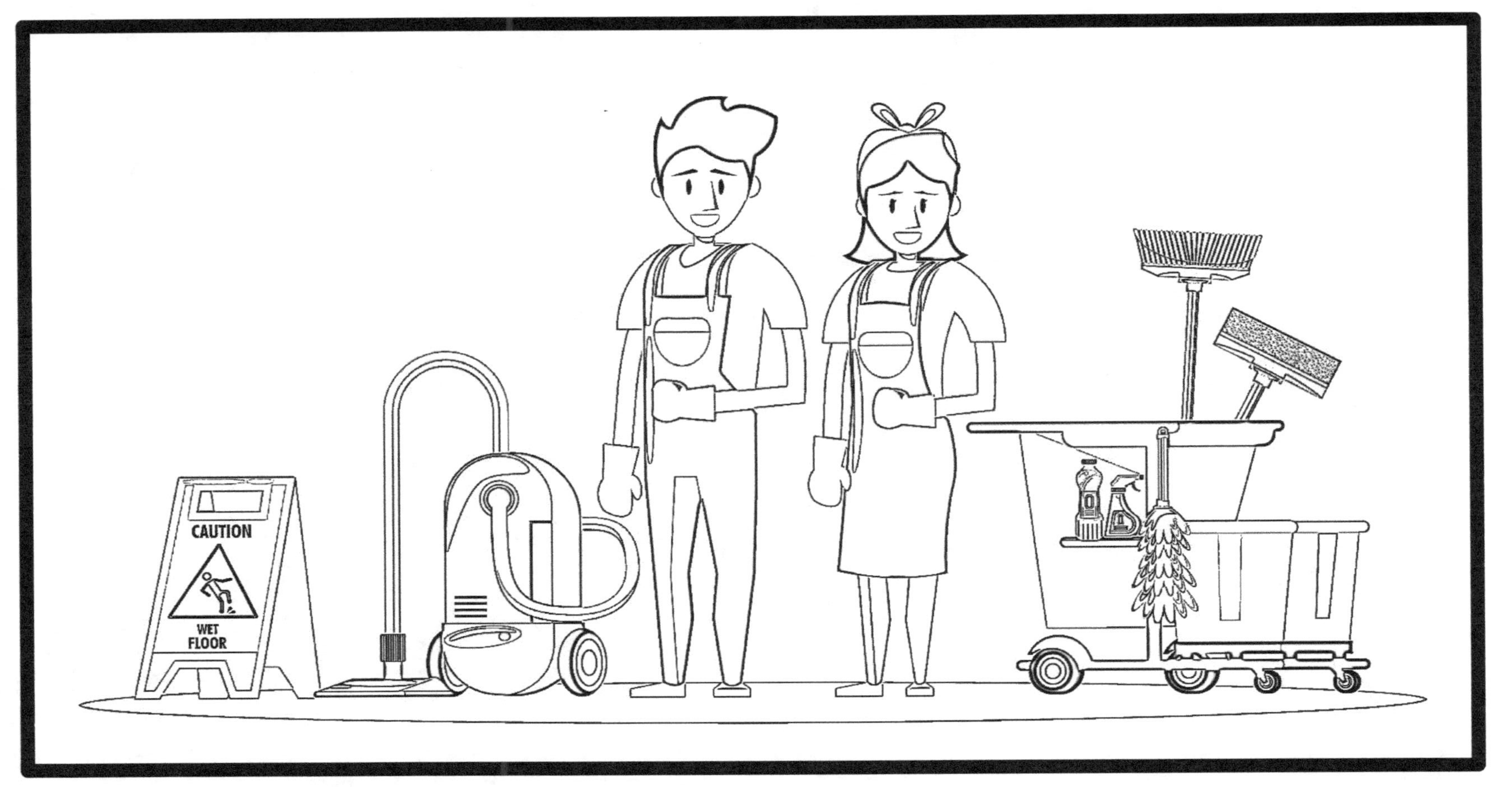

CAUTION
WET
FLOOR

Artist Name:______________________

Date:______________________

Title:______________________

Dedicated to:______________________

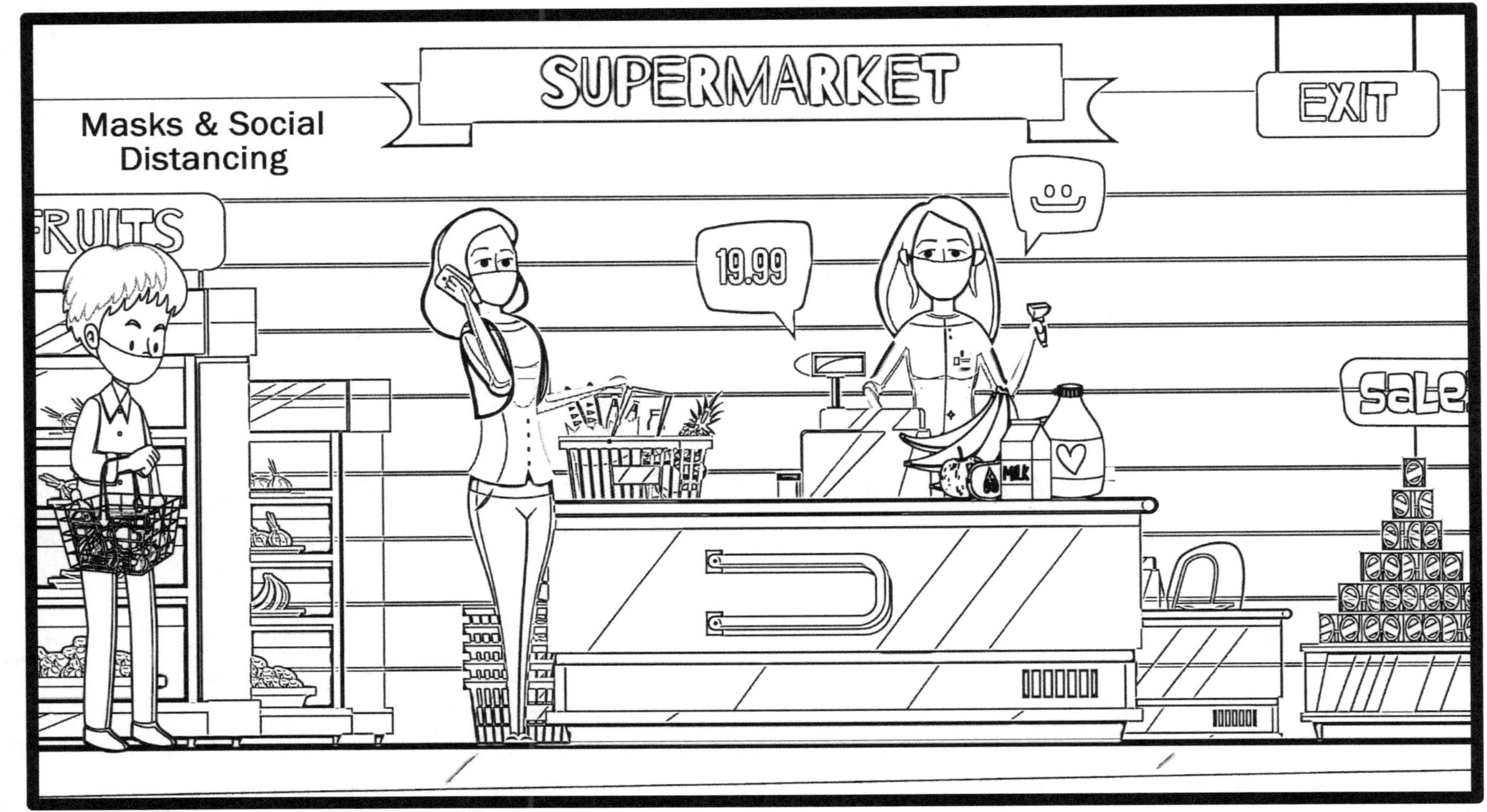

SUPERMARKET
EXIT
Masks & Social Distancing
FRUITS
19.99
SALE
MILK

Artist Name:

Date:

Title:

Dedicated to:

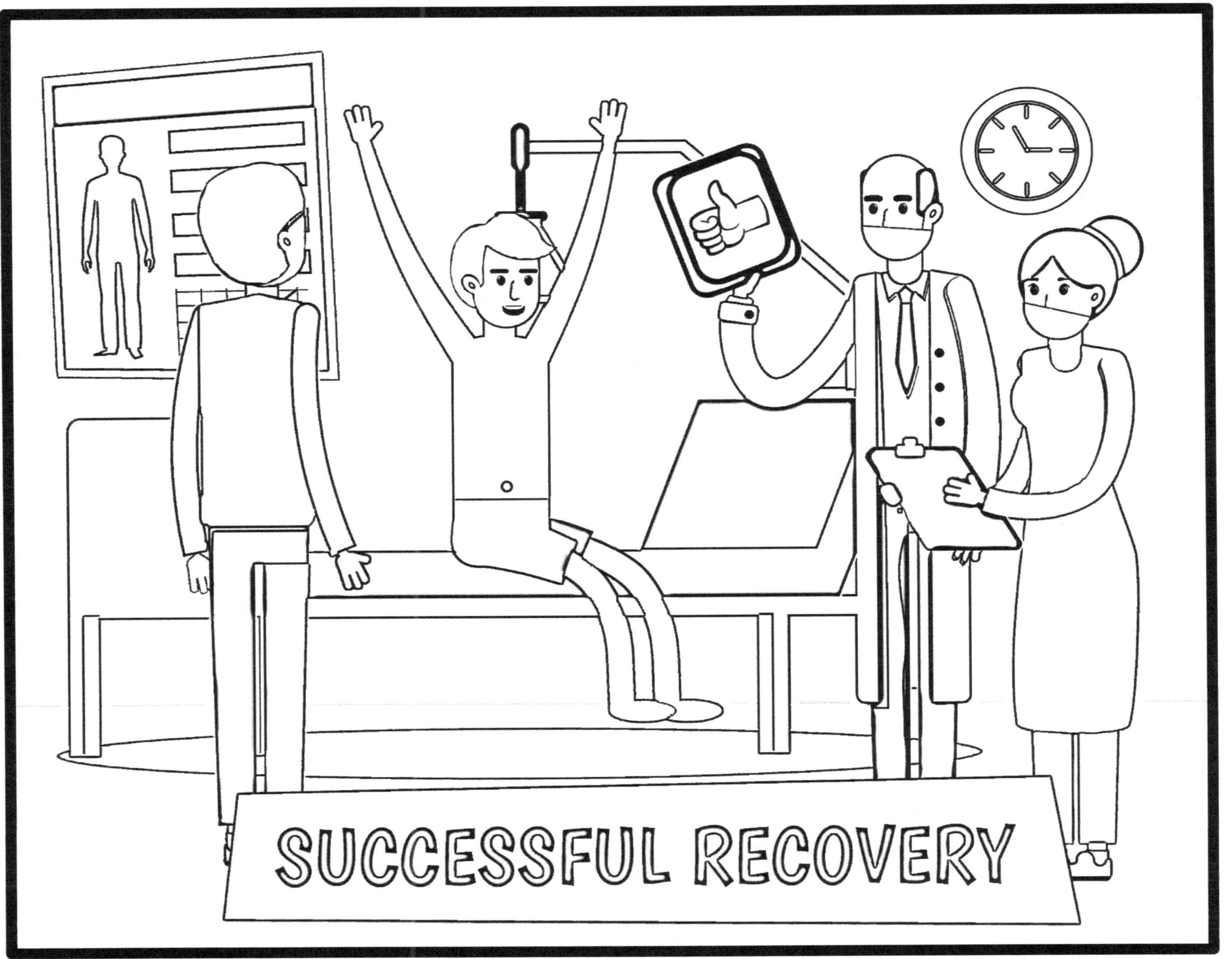

SUCCESSFUL RECOVERY

Artist Name:_______________________

Date:_______________________

Title:_______________________

Dedicated to:_______________________

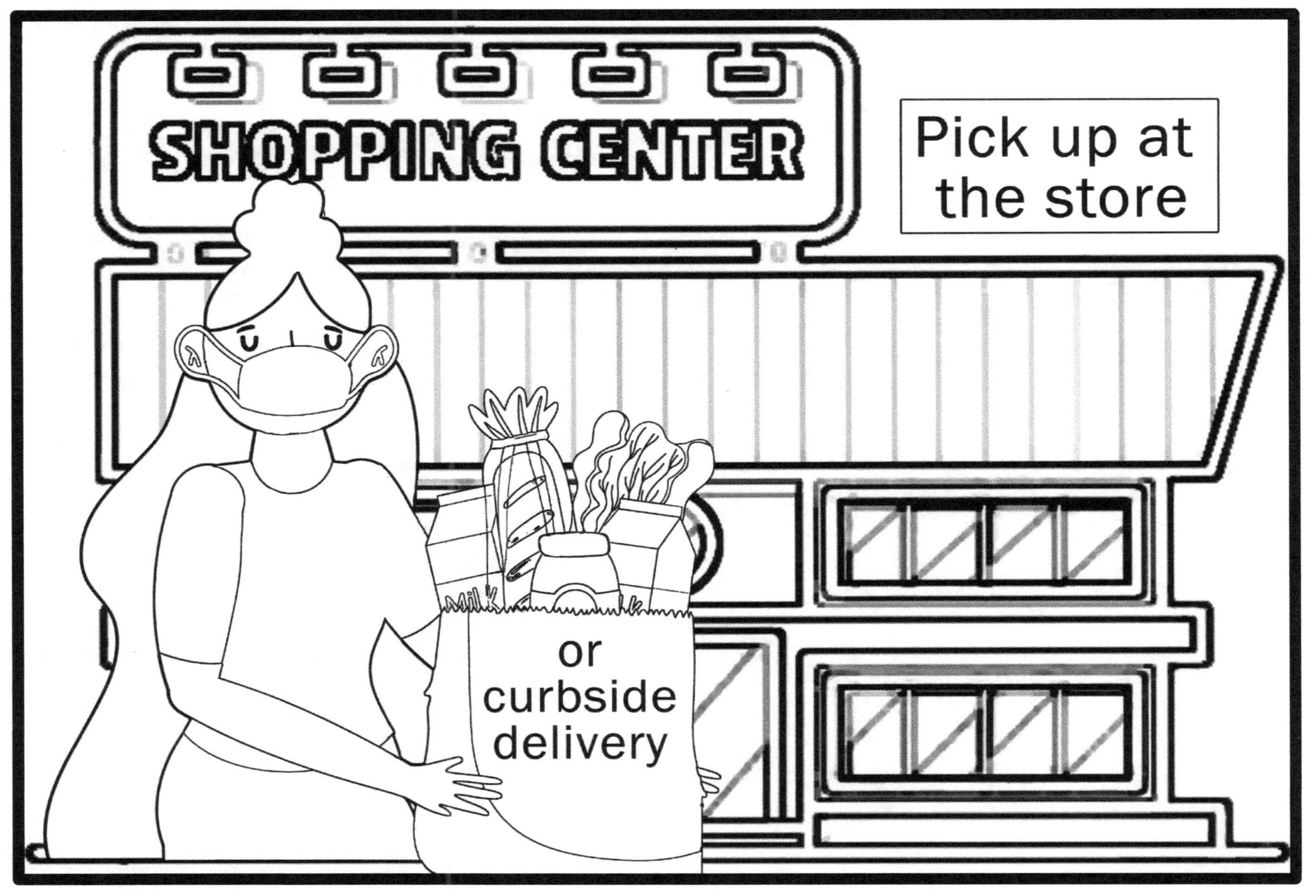

SHOPPING CENTER
Pick up at the store
Milk
or curbside delivery

Artist Name:_______________________

Date:_______________________

Title:_______________________

Dedicated to:_______________________

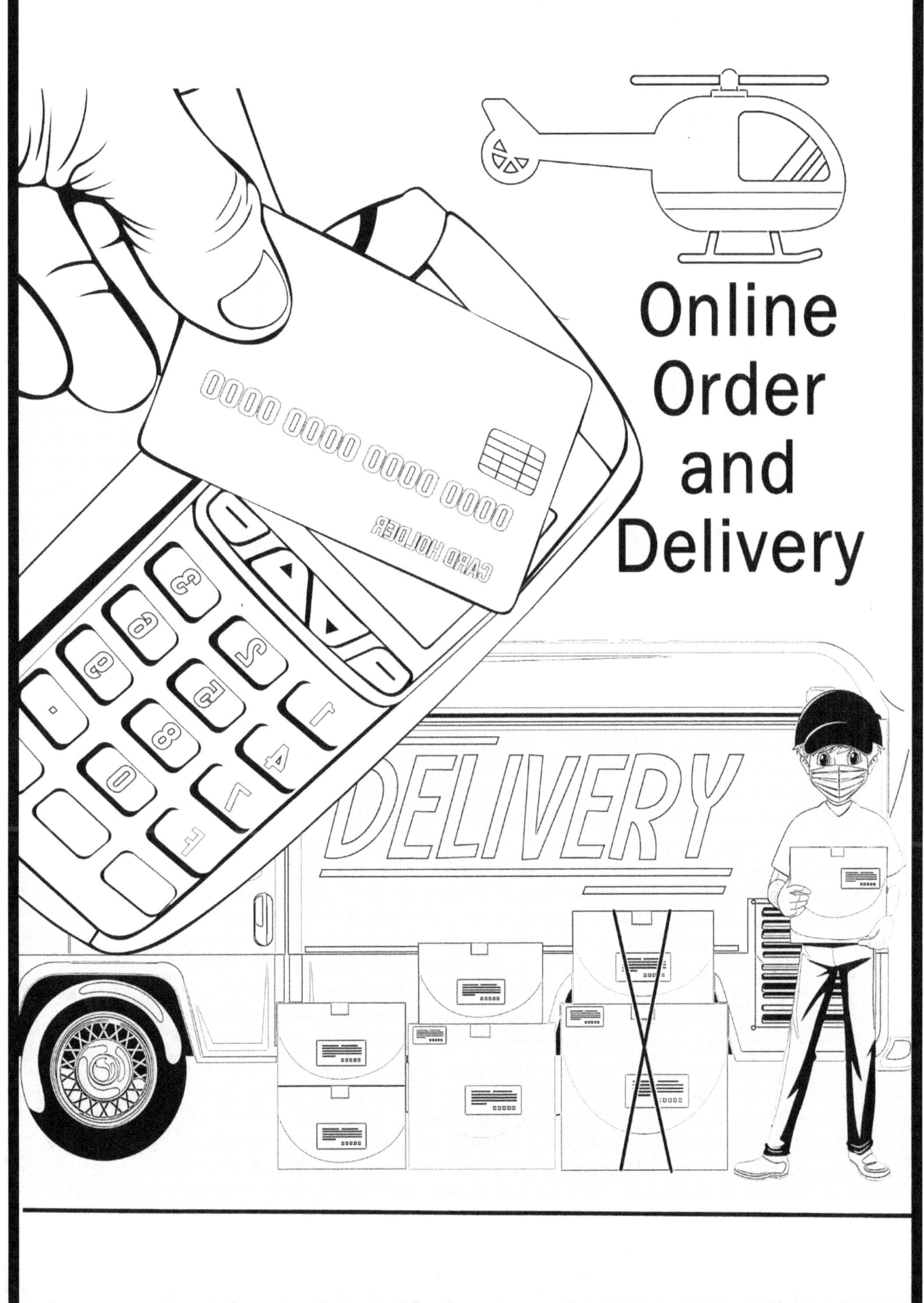

Online
Order
and
Delivery
DELIVERY
0000 0000 0000 0000
CARD HOLDER

Artist Name:

Date:

Title:

Dedicated to:

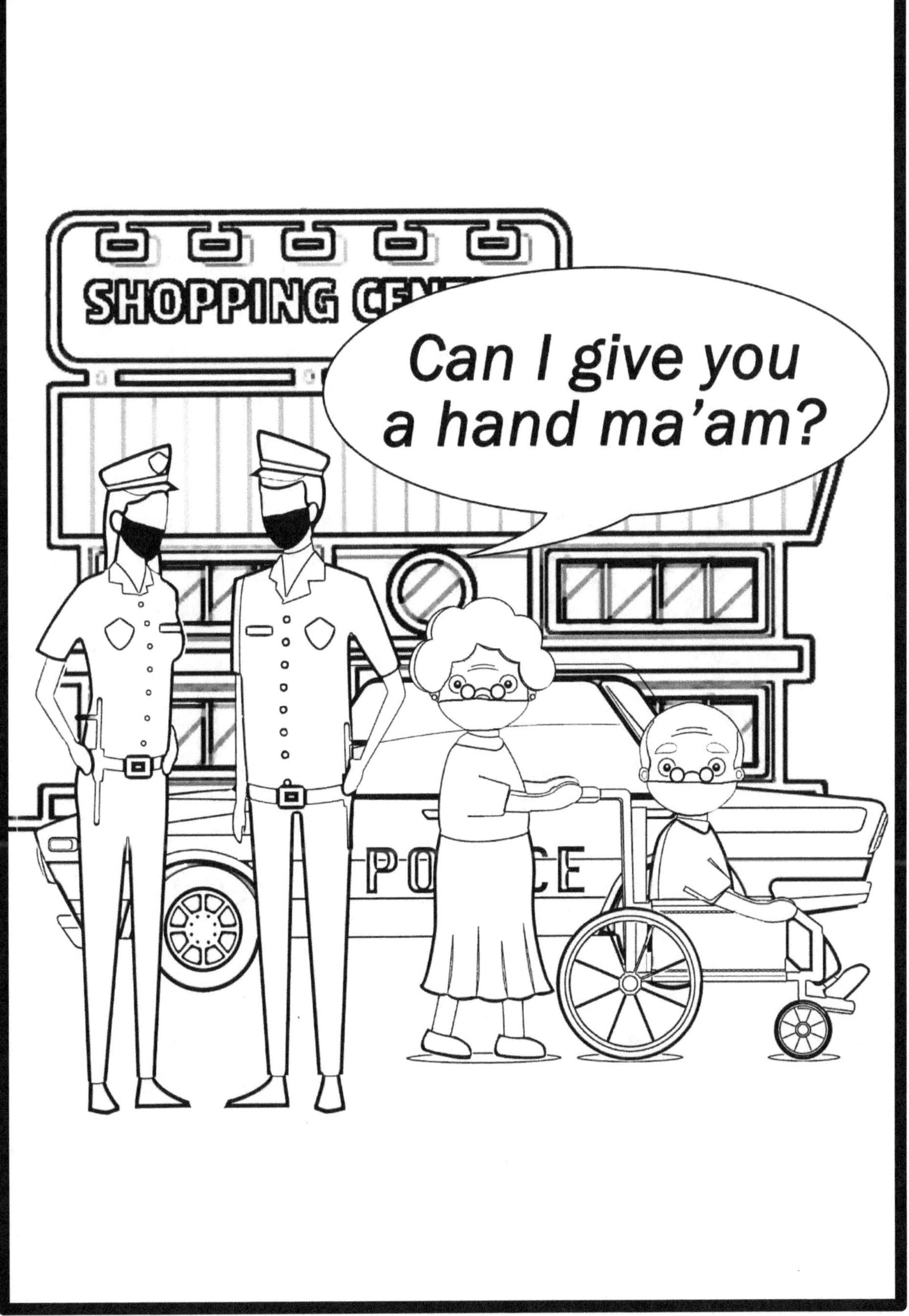

SHOPPING CENTER
Can I give you
a hand ma'am?
POLICE

Artist Name:

Date:

Title:

Dedicated to:

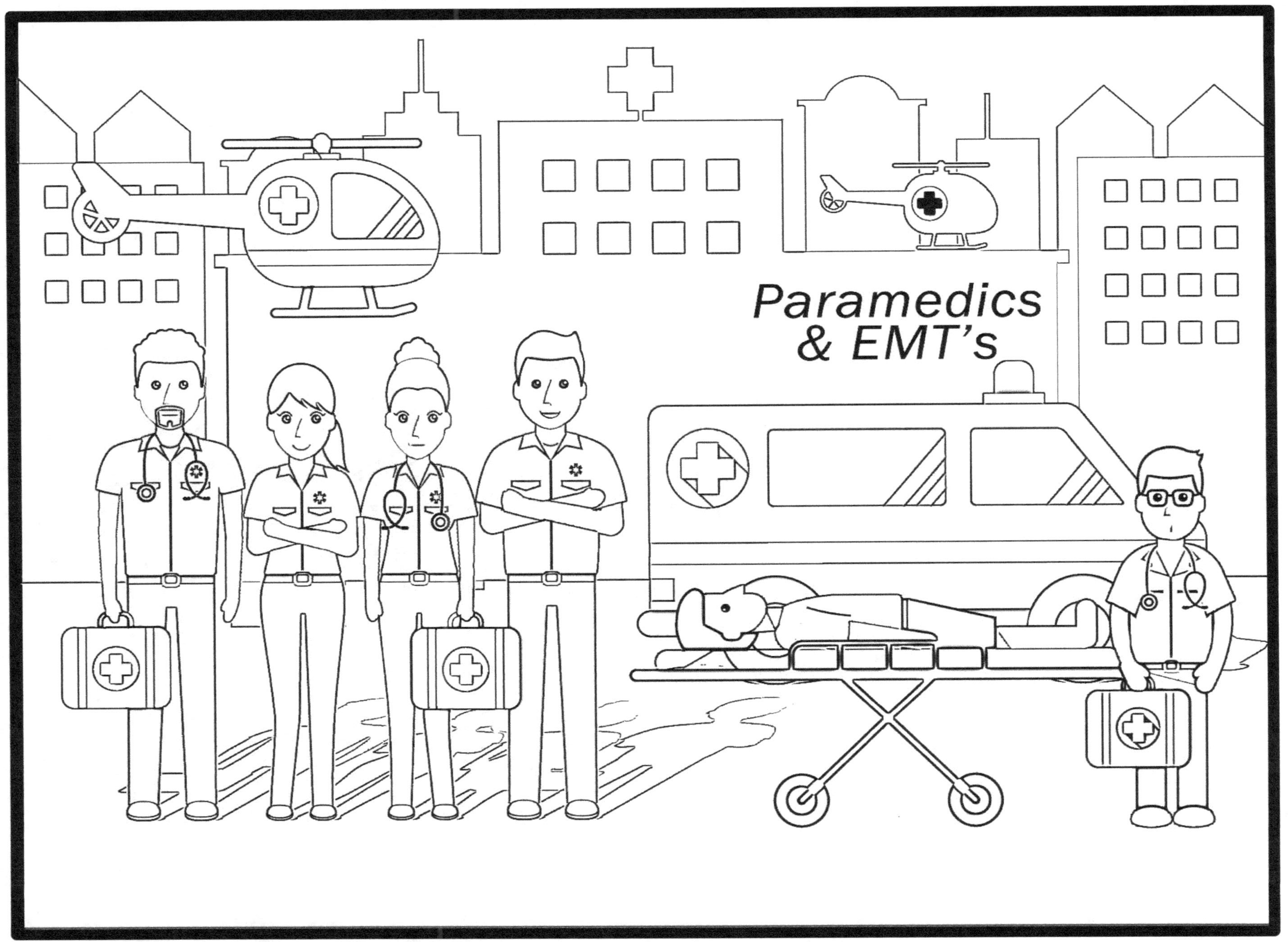

Paramedics
& EMT's

Artist Name: _______________

Date: _______________

Title: _______________

Dedicated to: _______________

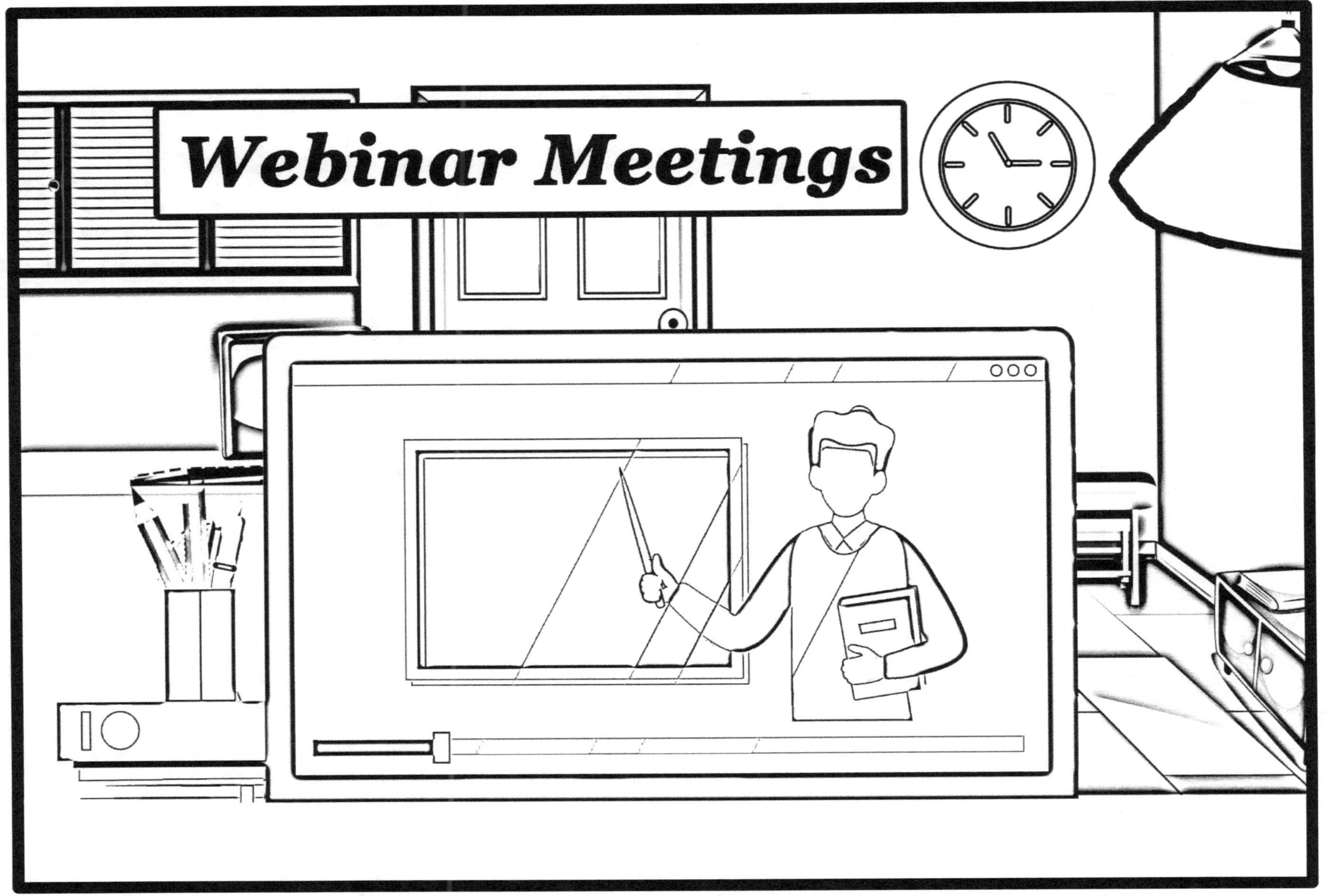

Webinar Meetings

Artist Name:_______________________

Date:_______________________

Title:_______________________

Dedicated to:_______________________

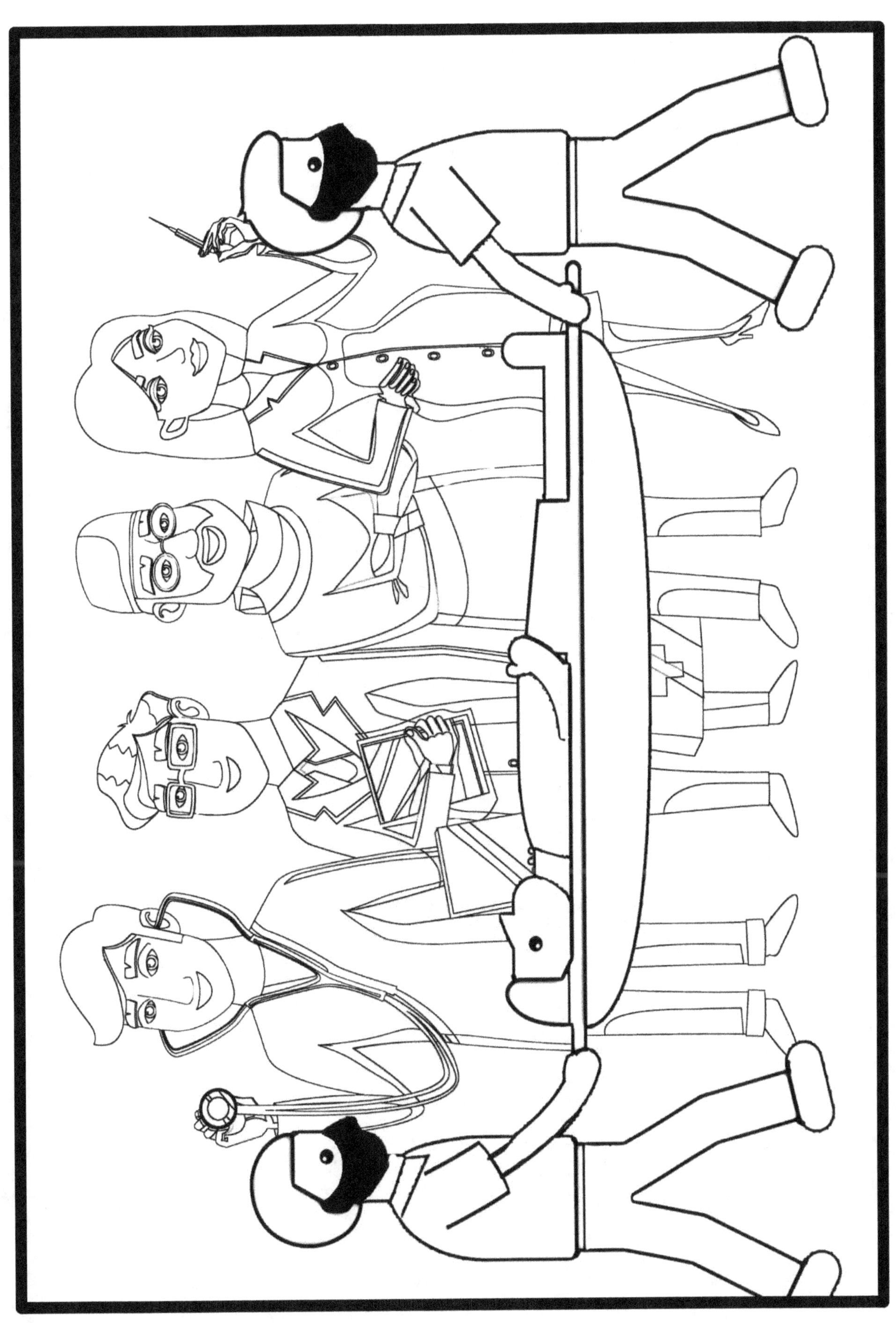

Artist Name:_______________

Date:_______________

Title:_______________

Dedicated to:_______________

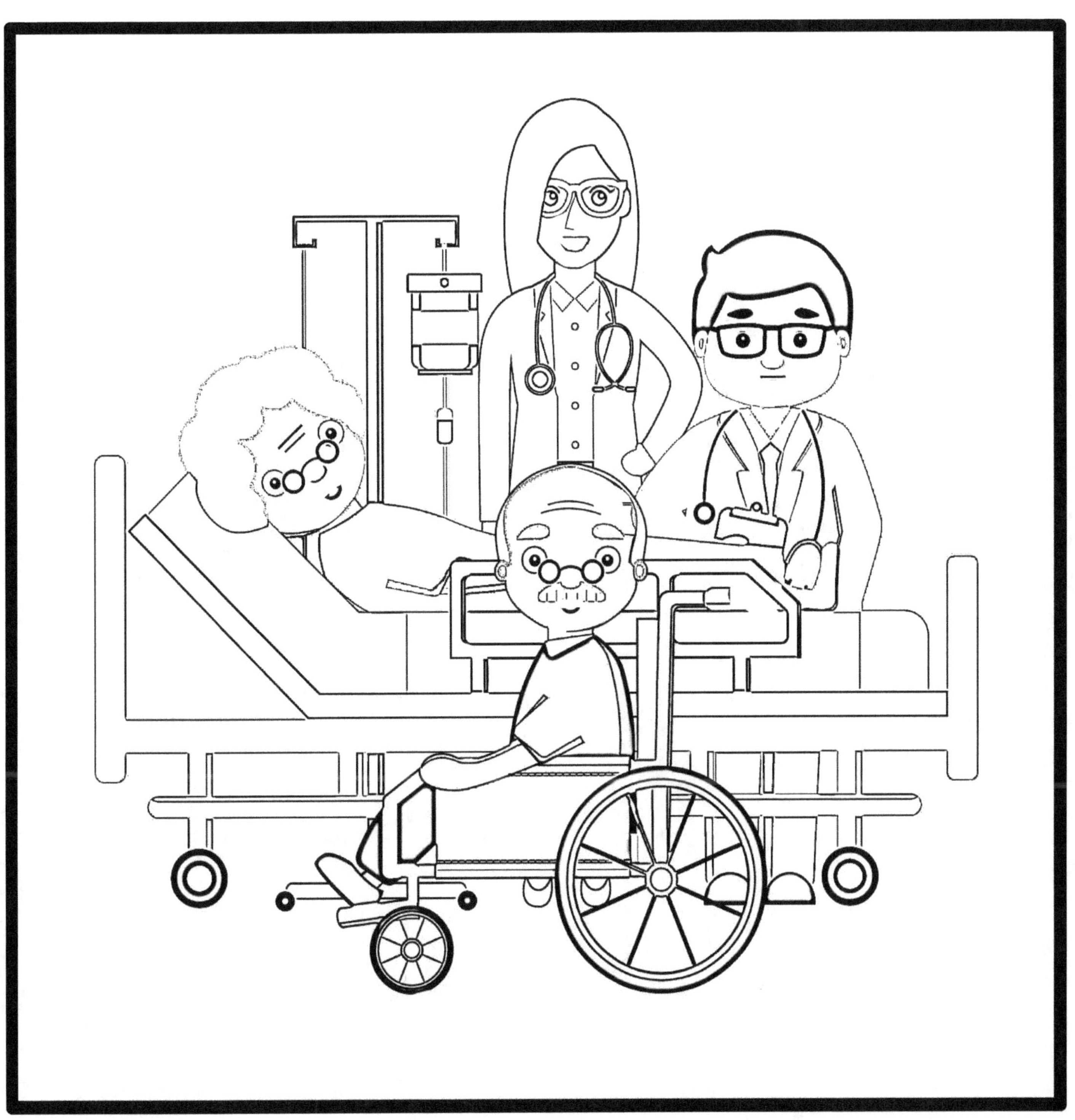

Artist Name:_______________________________

Date:_______________________________

Title:_______________________________

Dedicated to:_______________________________

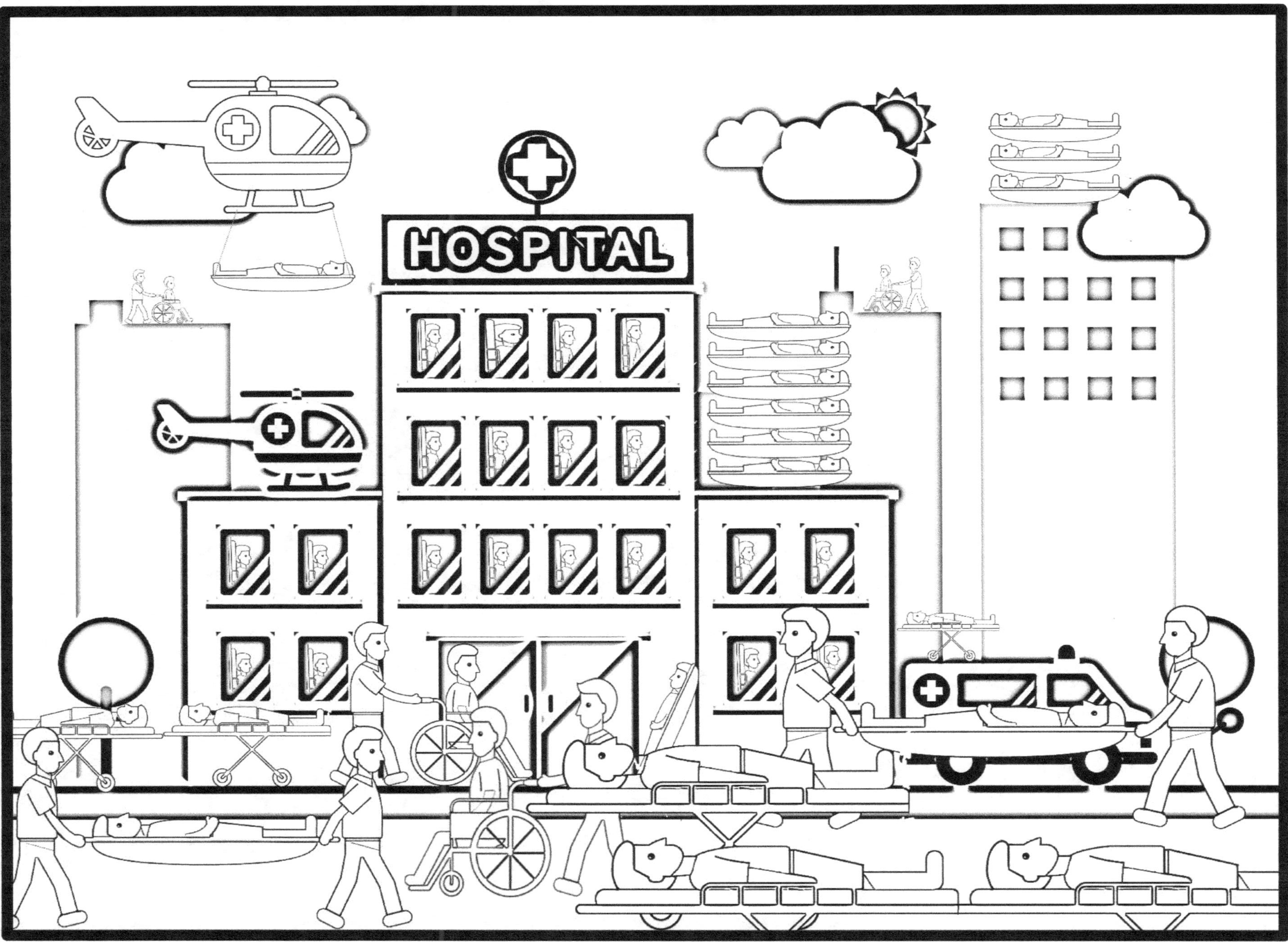
HOSPITAL

Artist Name:_______________________

Date:_______________________

Title:_______________________

Dedicated to:_______________________

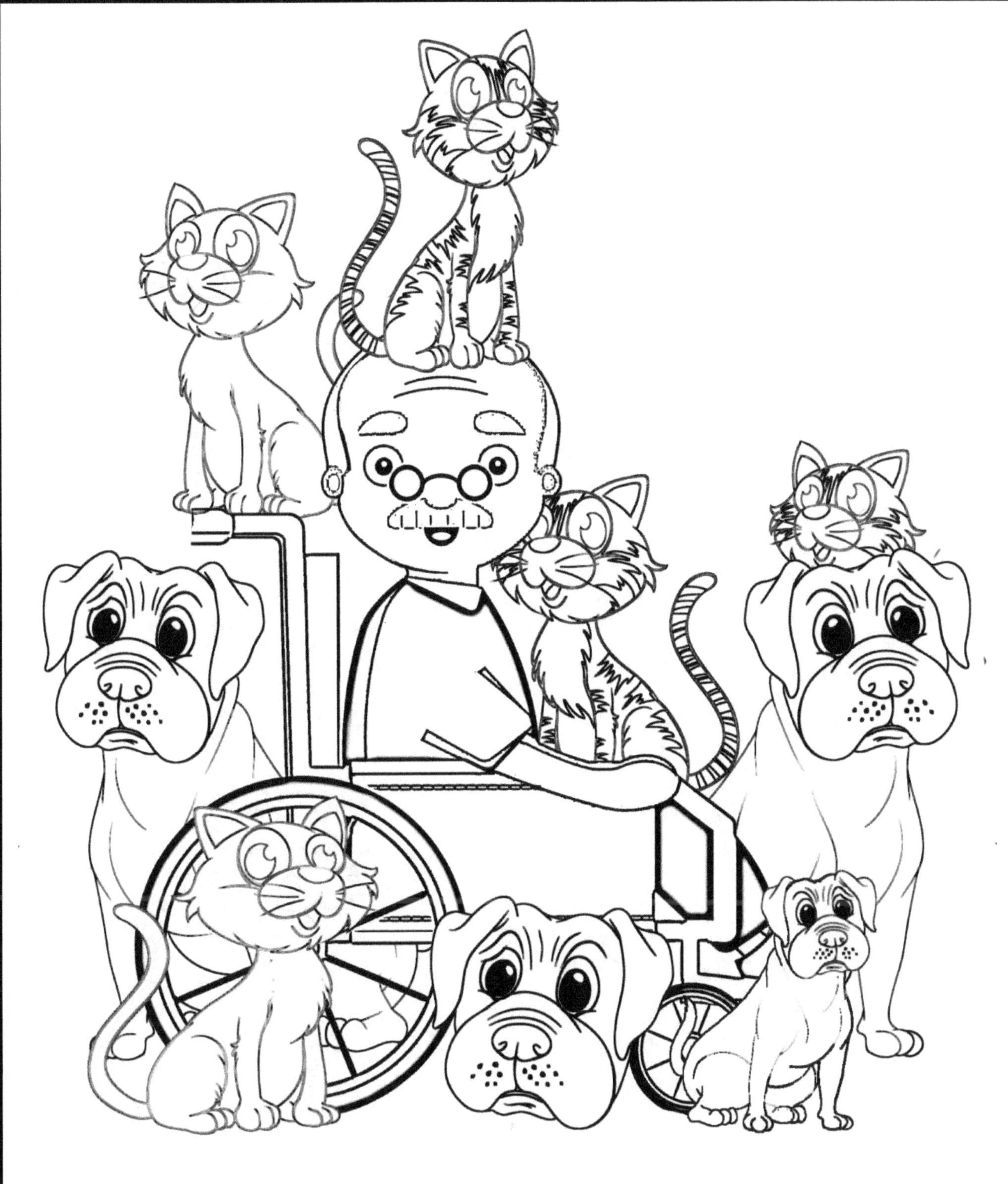

I have plenty of friends.

Artist Name:

Date:

Title:

Dedicated to:

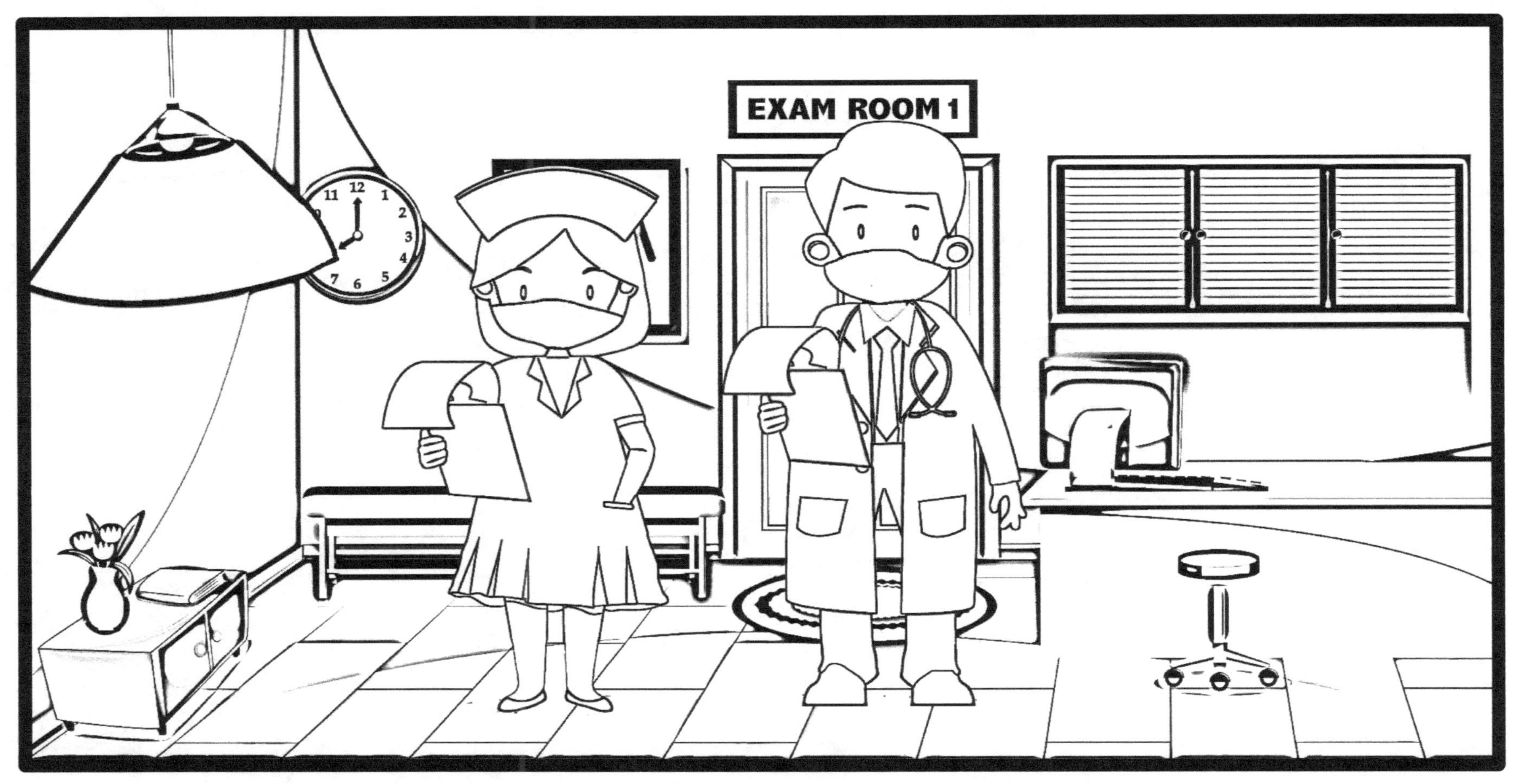

EXAM ROOM 1

Artist Name:_________________

Date:_________________

Title:_________________

Dedicated to:_________________

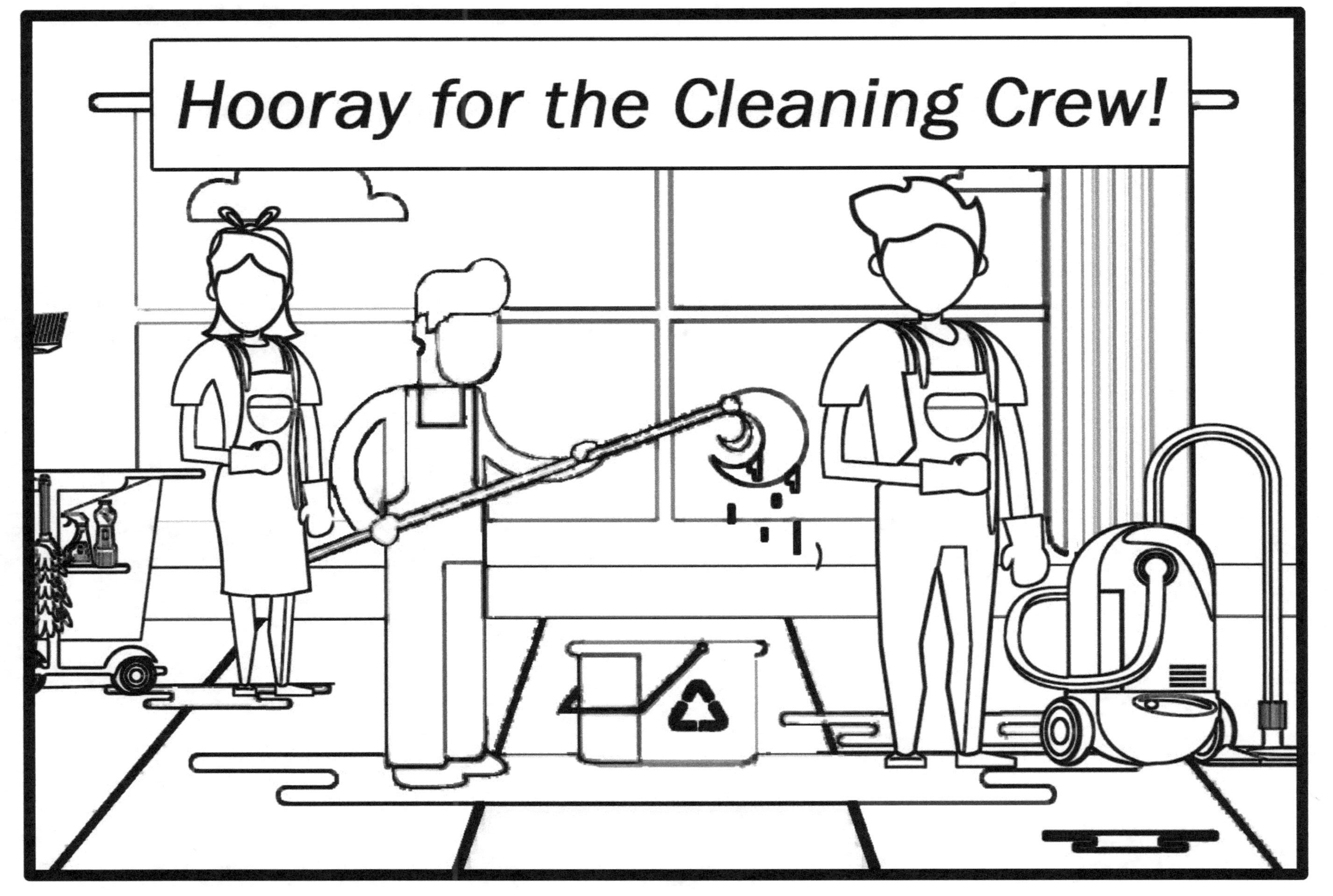

Hooray for the Cleaning Crew!

Artist Name:

Date:

Title:

Dedicated to:

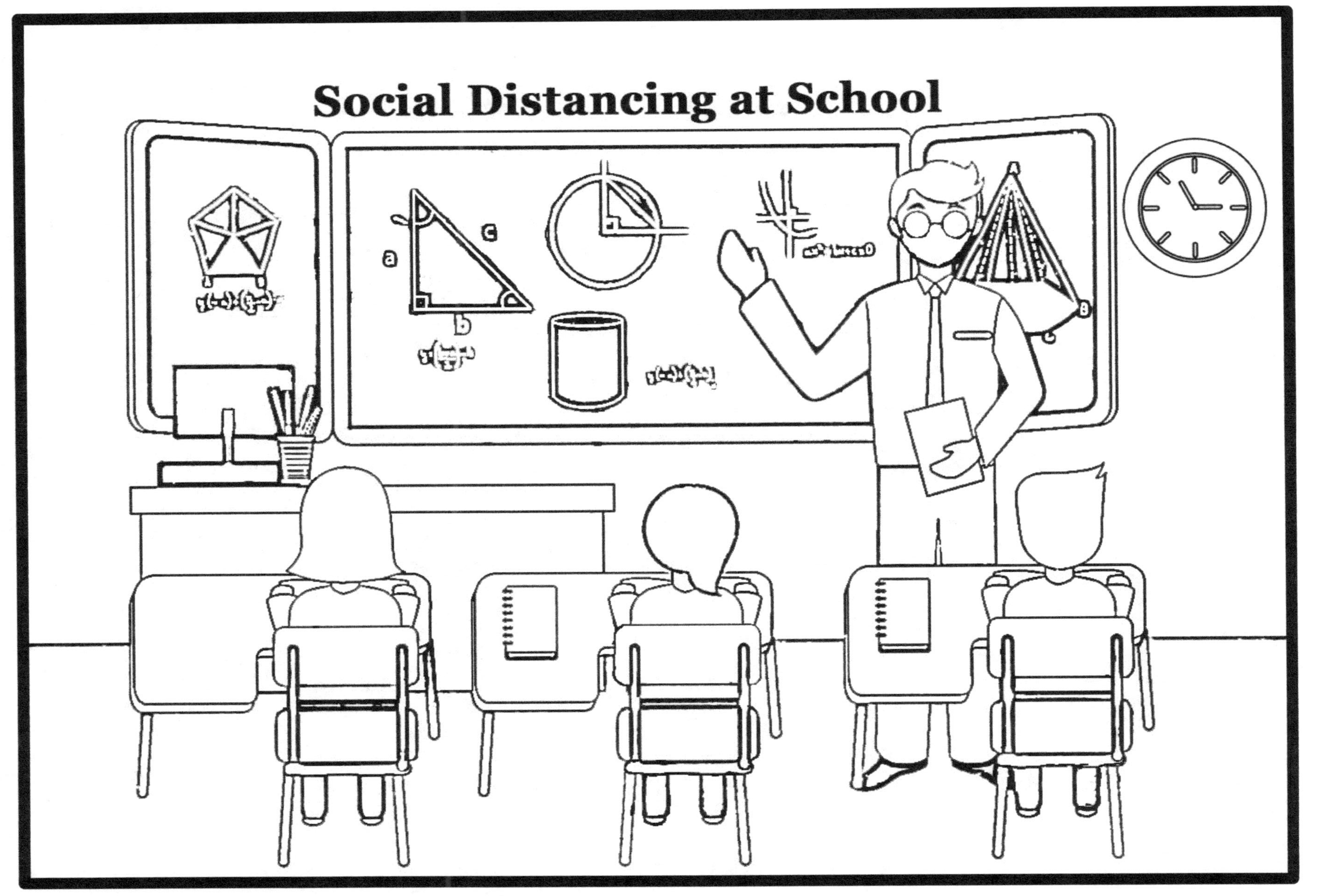

Social Distancing at School

Artist Name:____________________

Date:____________________

Title:____________________

Dedicated to:____________________

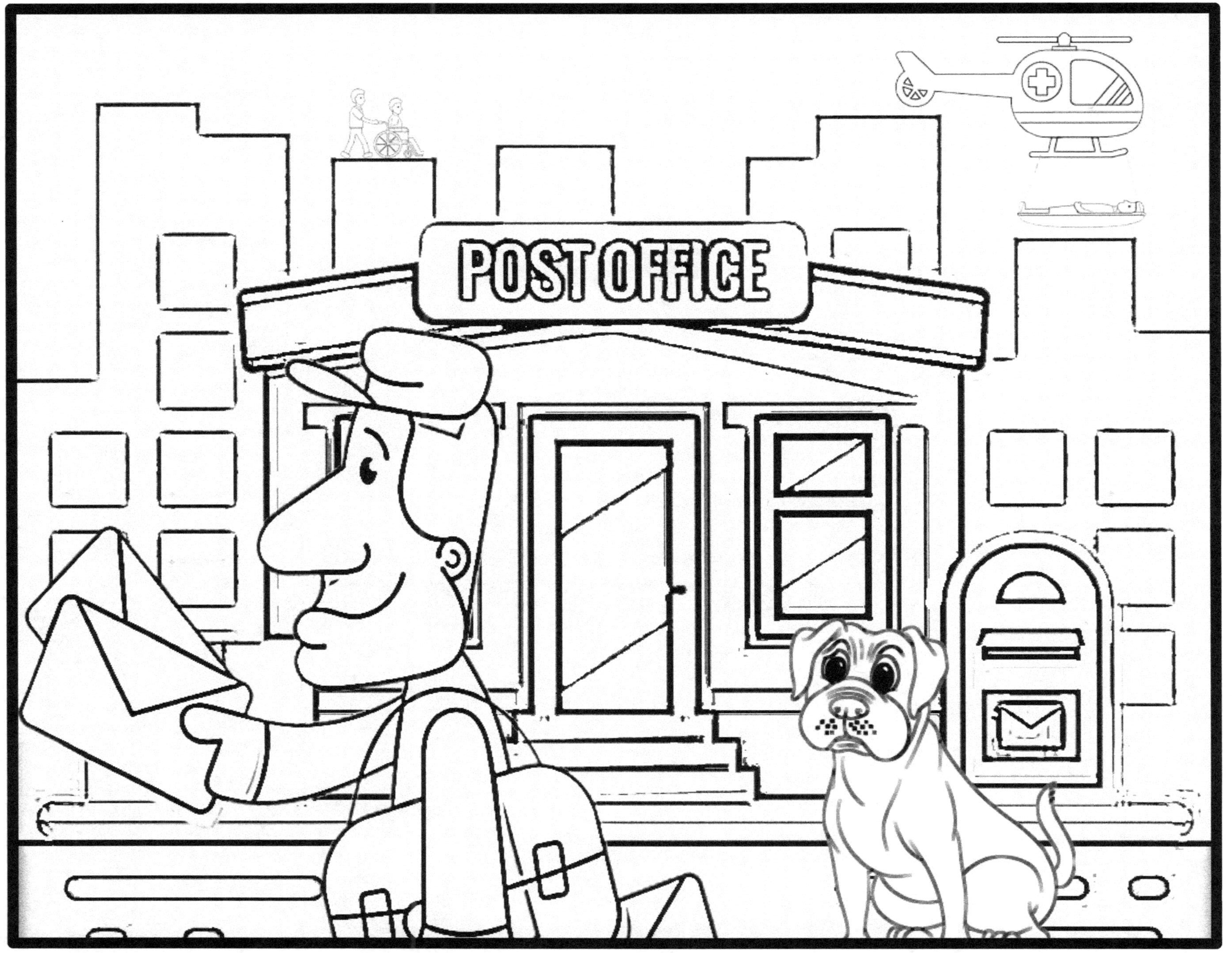

POST OFFICE

Artist Name:______________________

Date:______________________

Title:______________________

Dedicated to:______________________

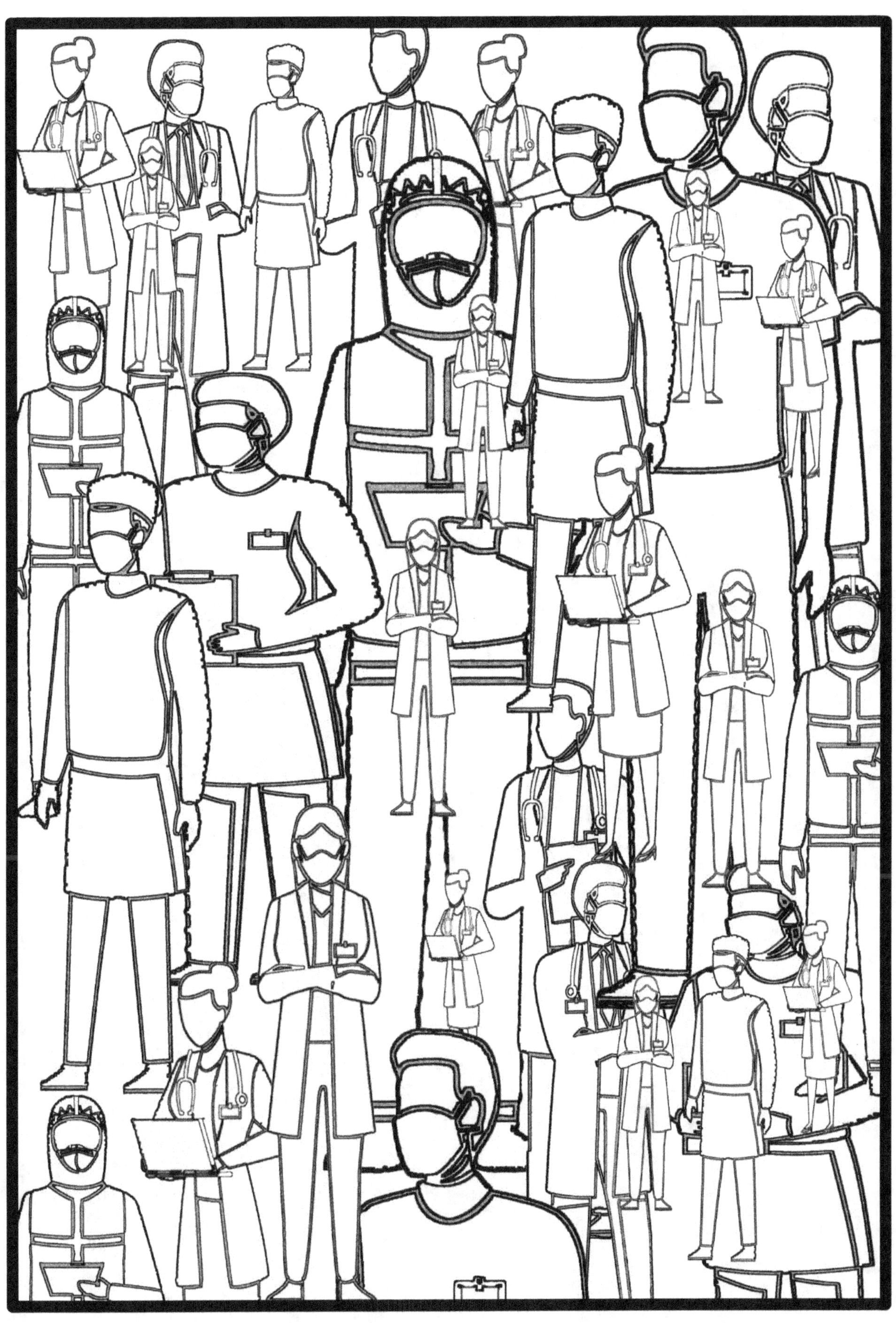

Artist Name:

Date:

Title:

Dedicated to:

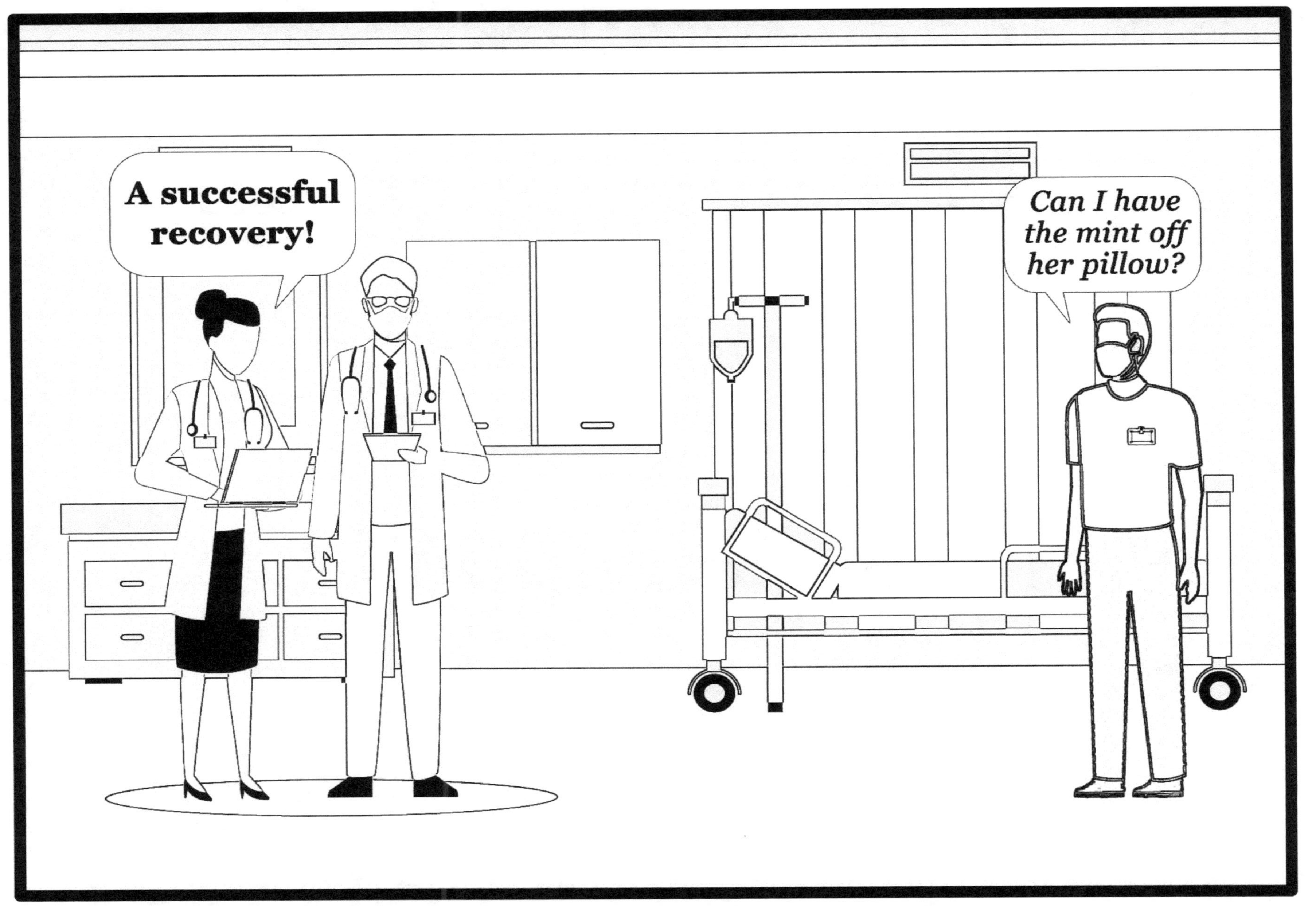

A successful recovery!
Can I have the mint off her pillow?

Artist Name:________________________

Date:________________________

Title:________________________

Dedicated to:________________________

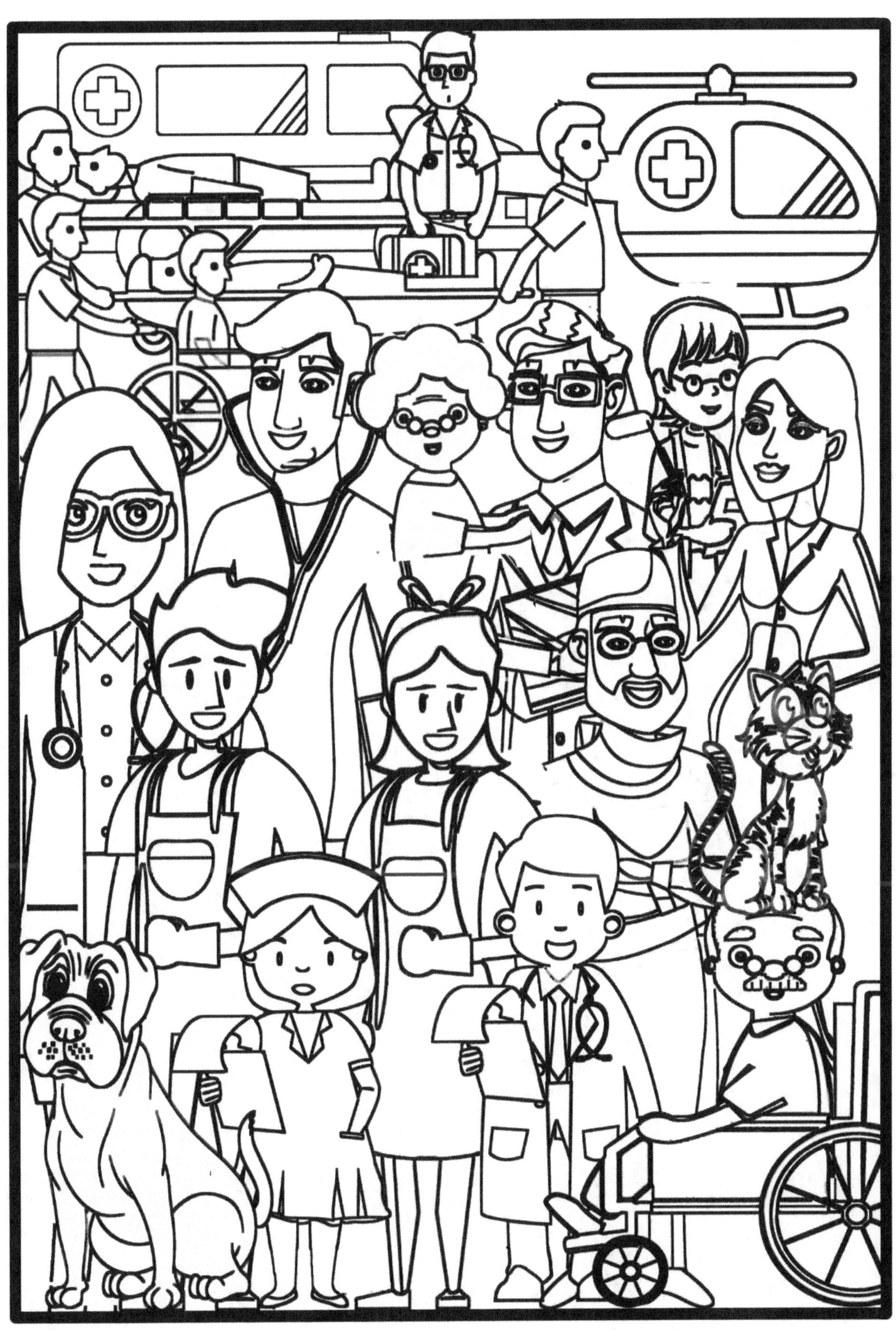

Artist Name:_________________________________

Date:_________________________________

Title:_________________________________

Dedicated to:_________________________________

Pharmacist

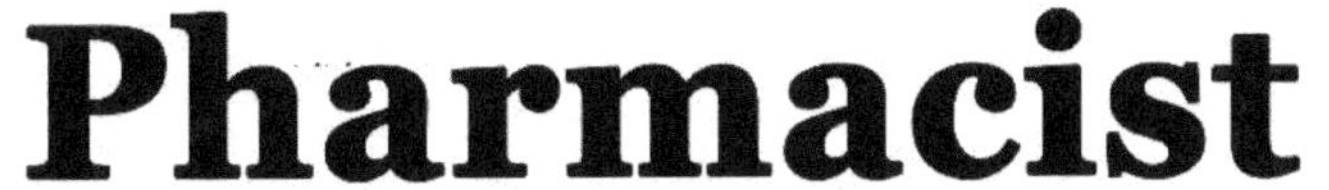

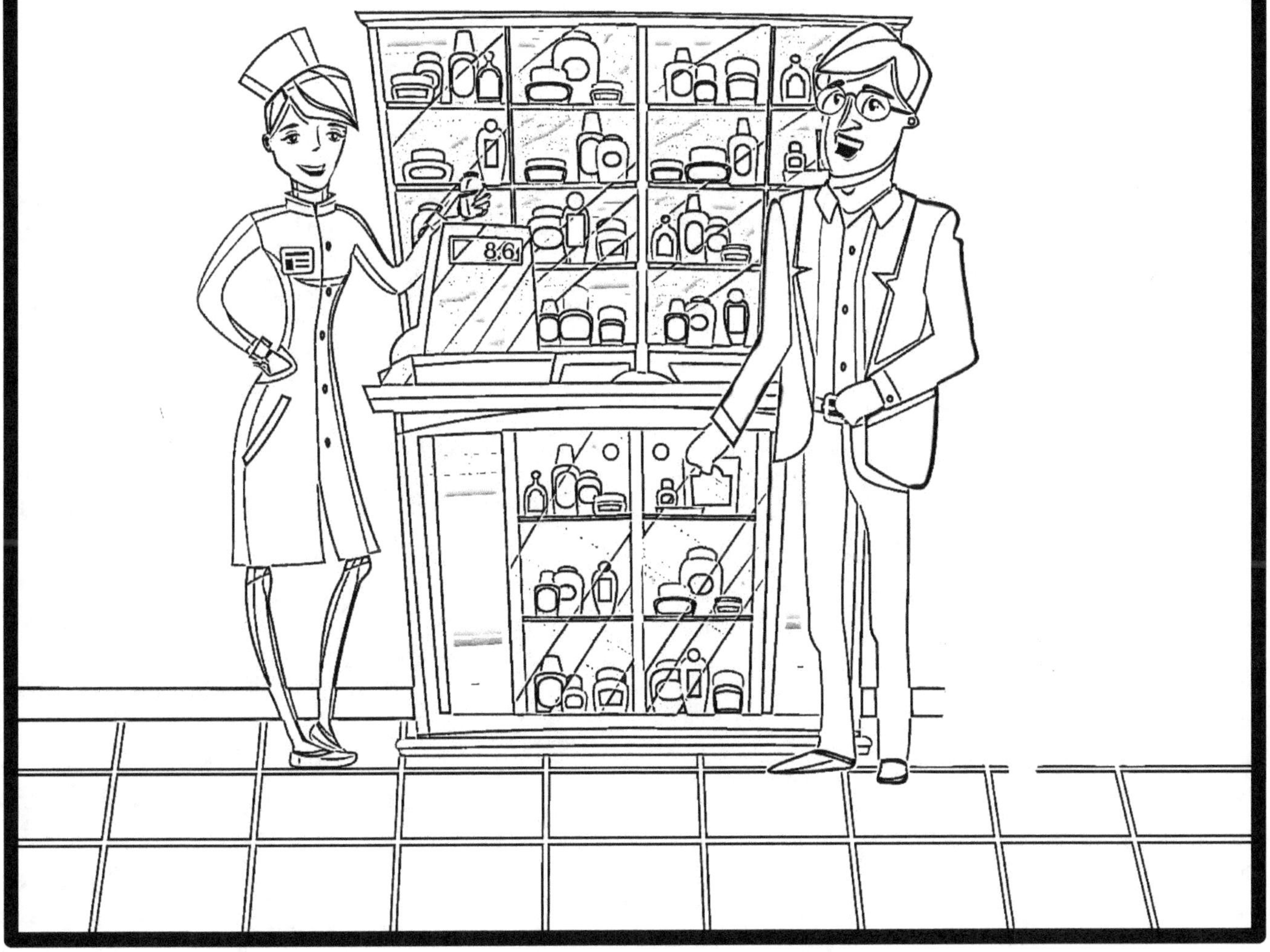

Artist Name:_______________________

Date:_______________________

Title:_______________________

Dedicated to:_______________________

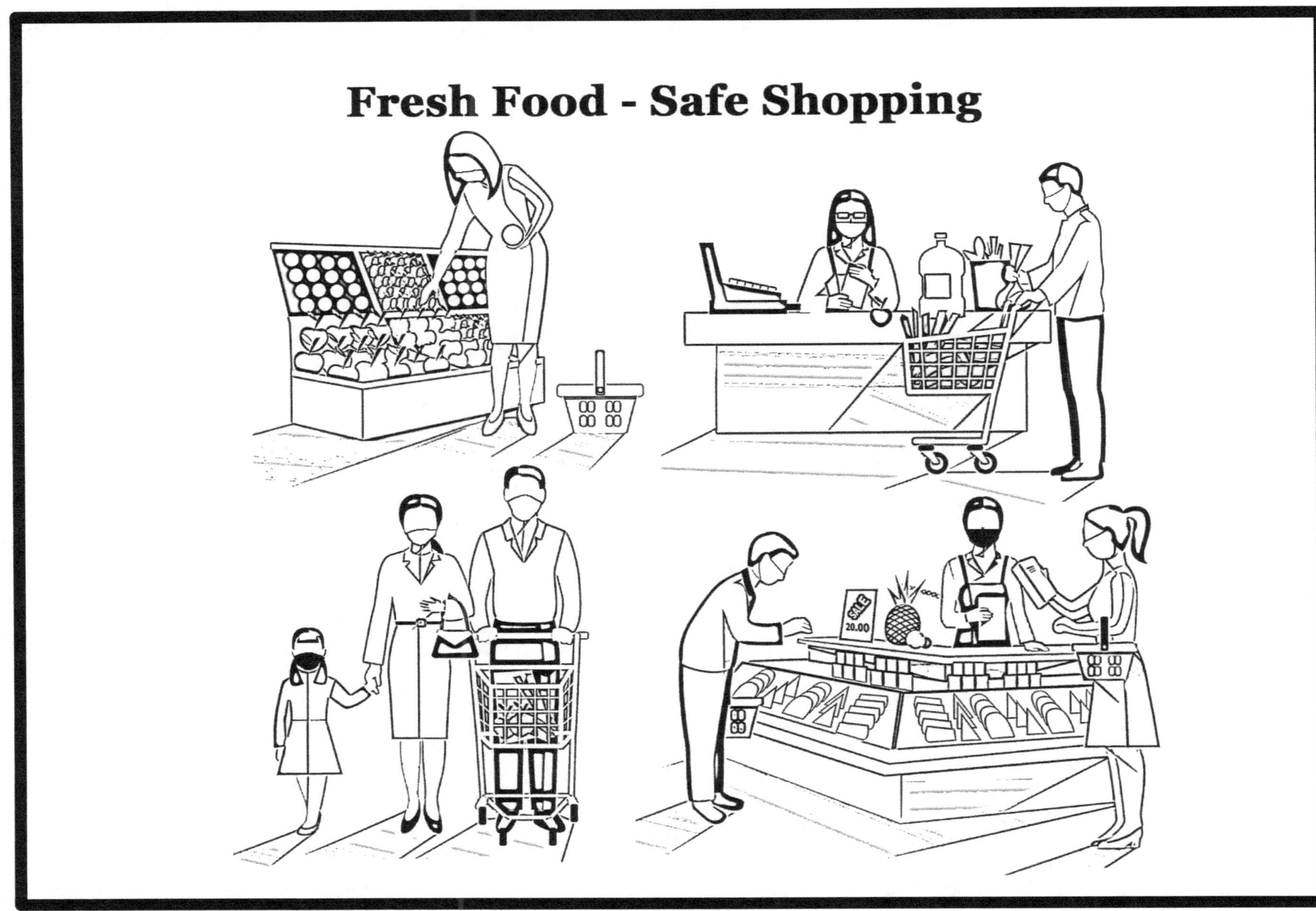

Fresh Food - Safe Shopping
SALE
20.00

Artist Name: _______________________

Date: _______________________

Title: _______________________

Dedicated to: _______________________

PIZZA! The Cure? Could be...

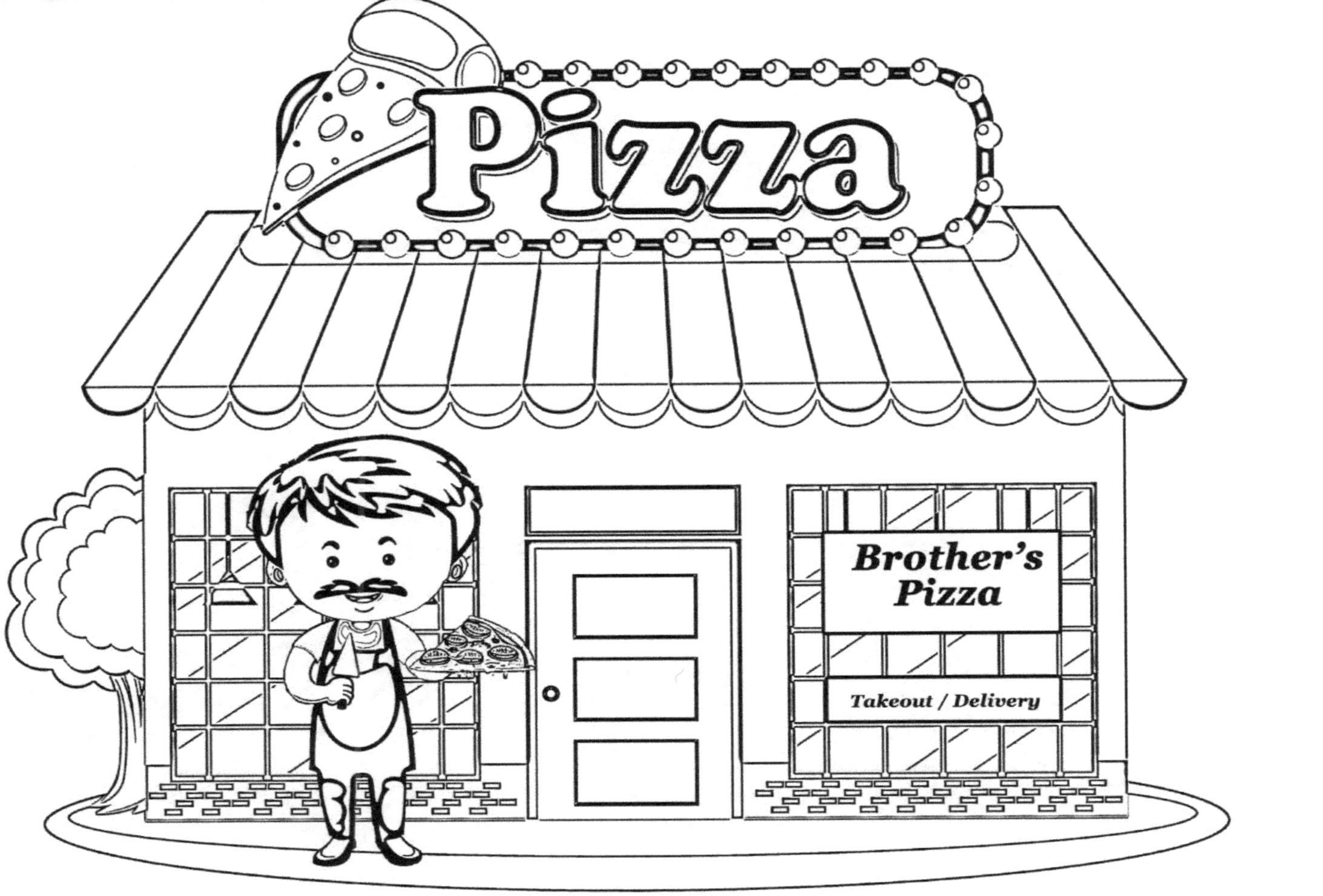

Artist Name:_______________________

Date:_______________________

Title:_______________________

Dedicated to:_______________________

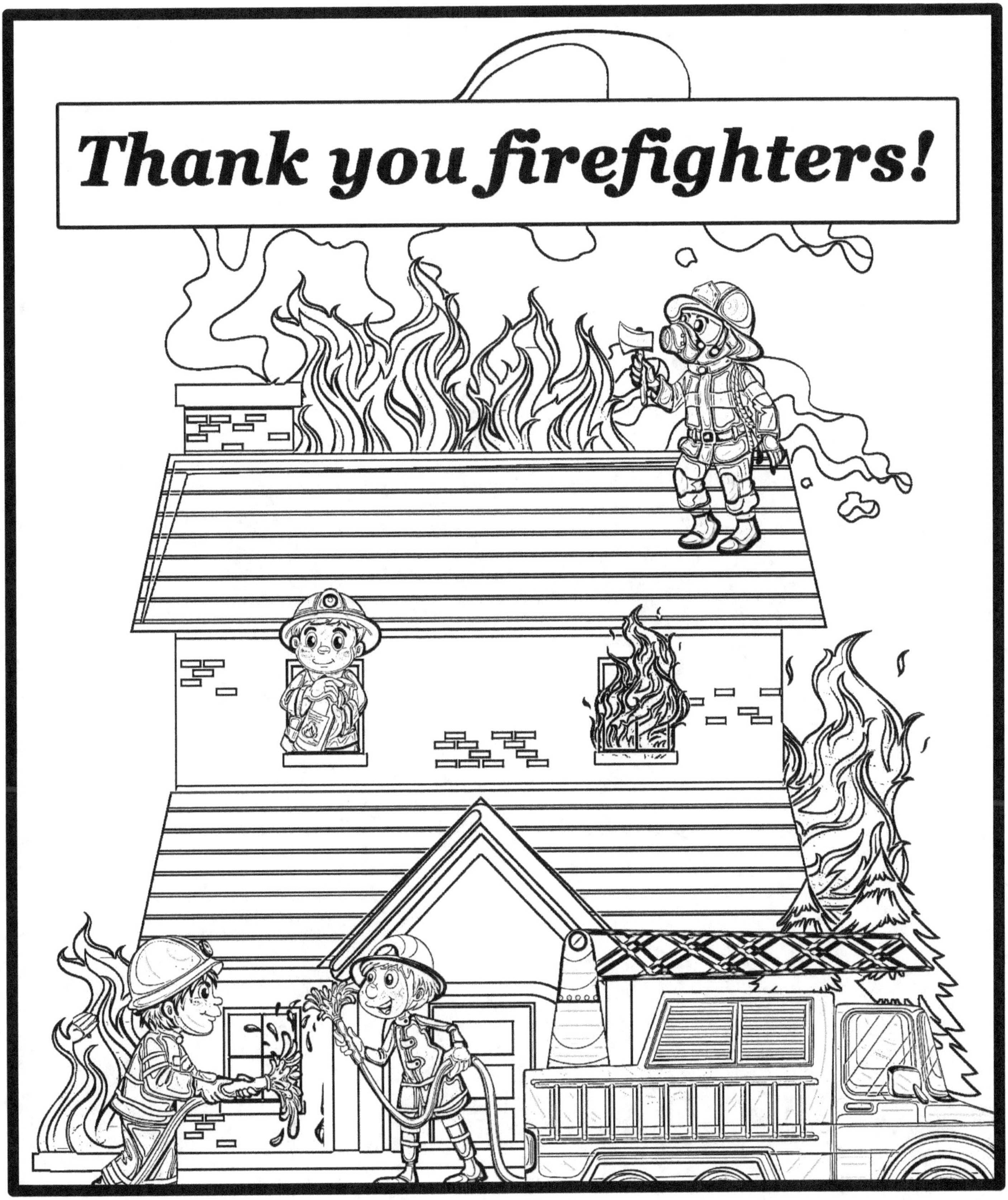

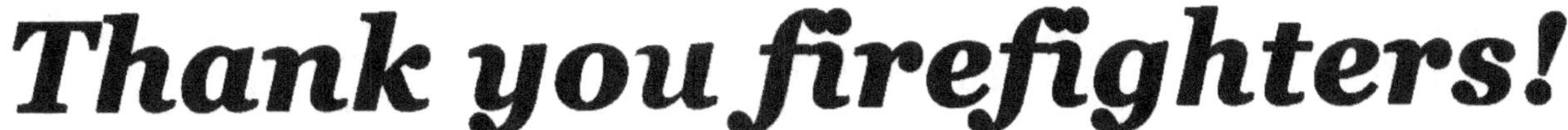
Thank you firefighters!

Artist Name: ___________________________

Date: ___________________________

Title: ___________________________

Dedicated to: ___________________________

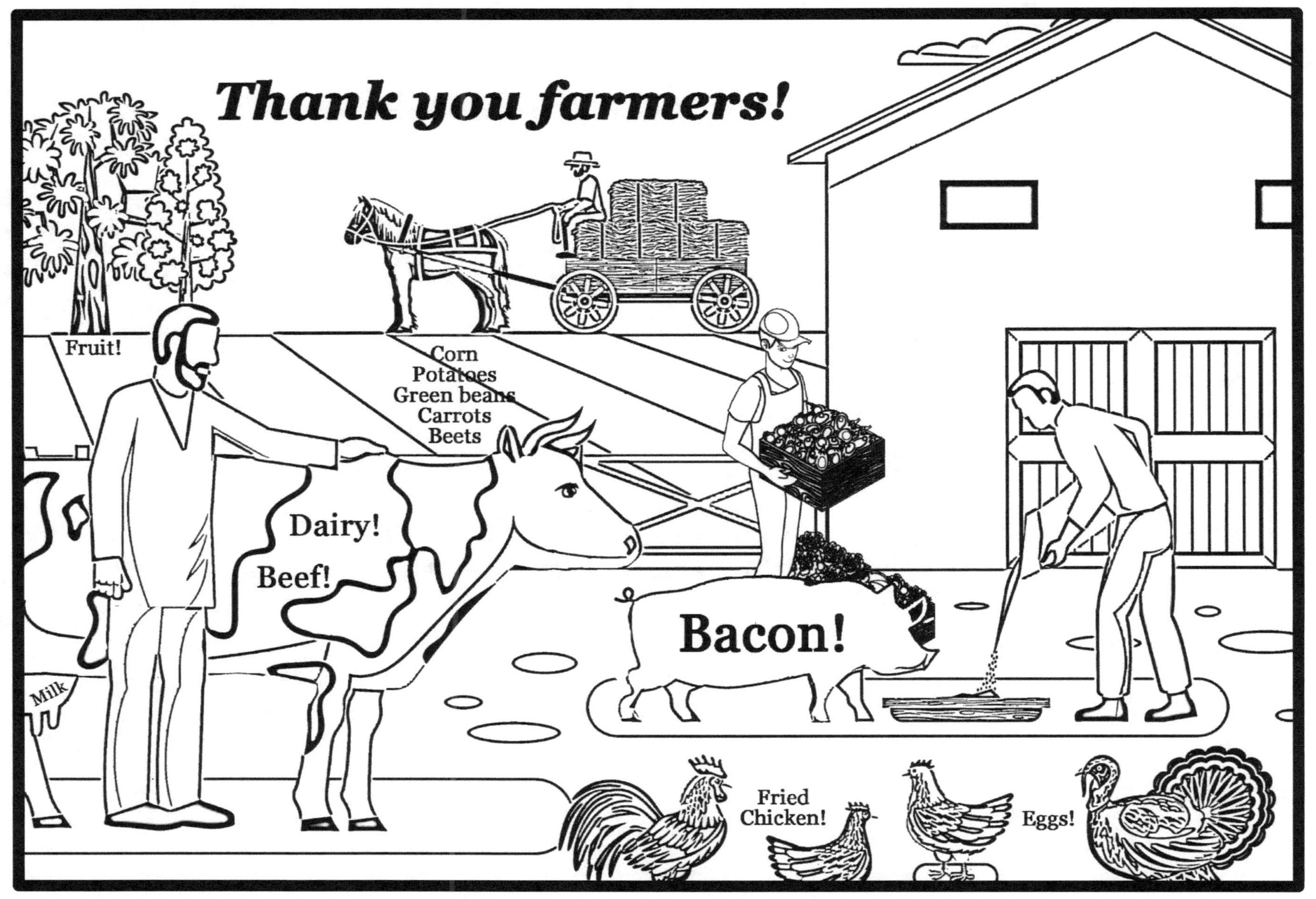

Thank you farmers!
Fruit!
Corn
Potatoes
Green beans
Carrots
Beets
Dairy!
Beef!
Milk
Bacon!
Fried Chicken!
Eggs!

Artist Name:_____________________

Date:_____________________

Title:_____________________

Dedicated to:_____________________

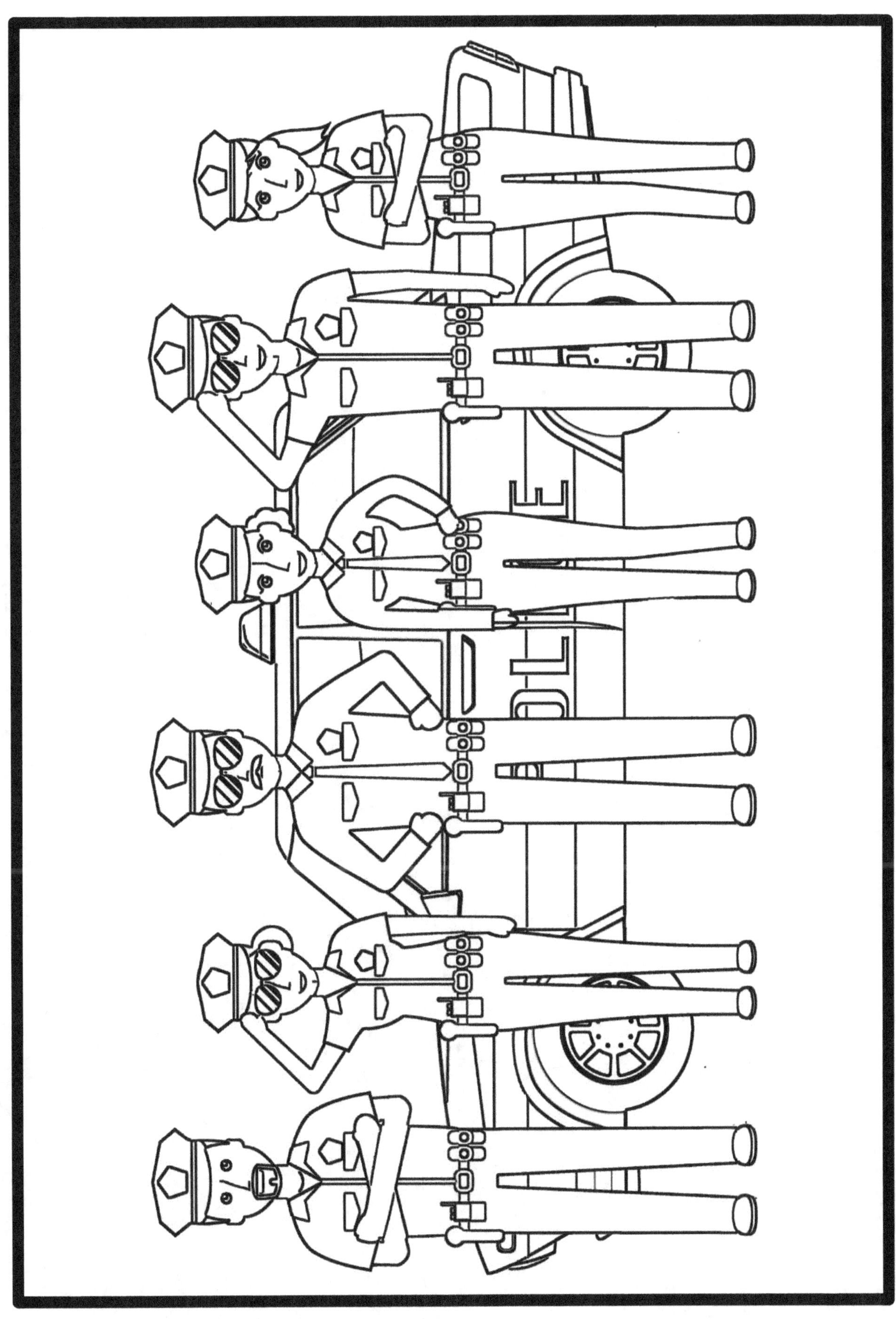

Artist Name:______________________

Date:______________________

Title:______________________

Dedicated to:______________________

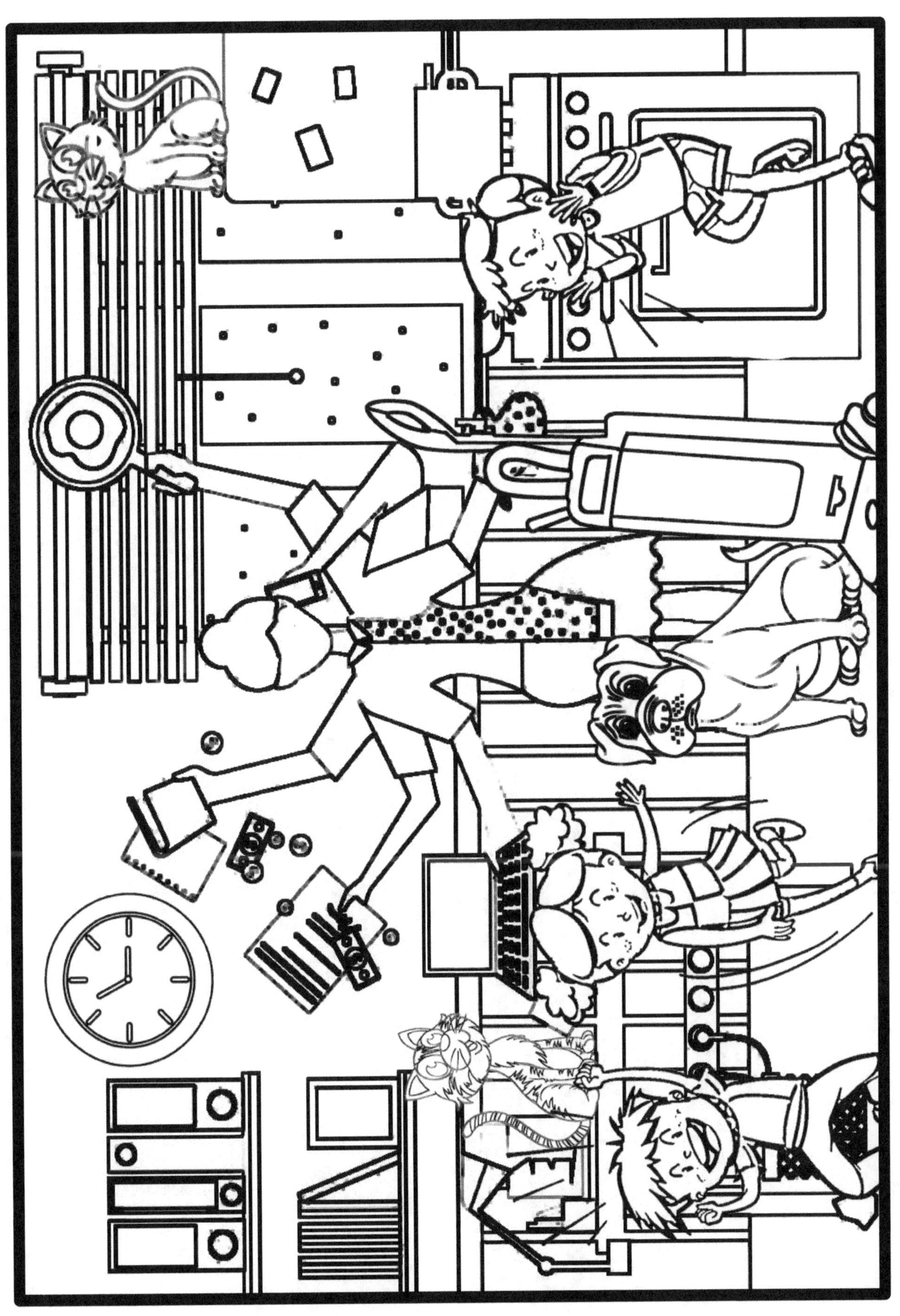

Artist Name:_____________________

Date:_____________________

Title:_____________________

Dedicated to:_____________________

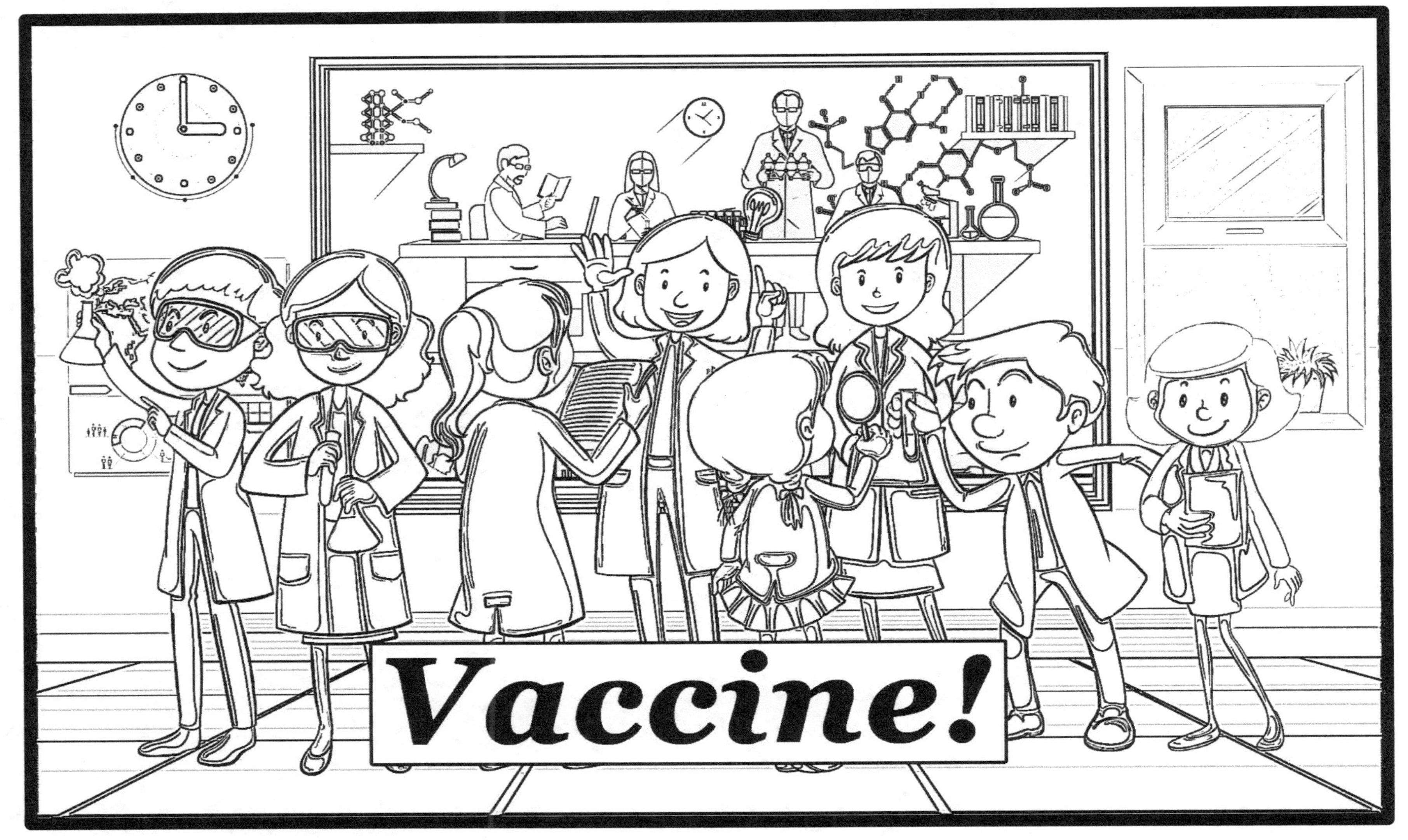

Vaccine!

Artist Name:_______________________

Date:_______________________

Title:_______________________

Dedicated to:_______________________

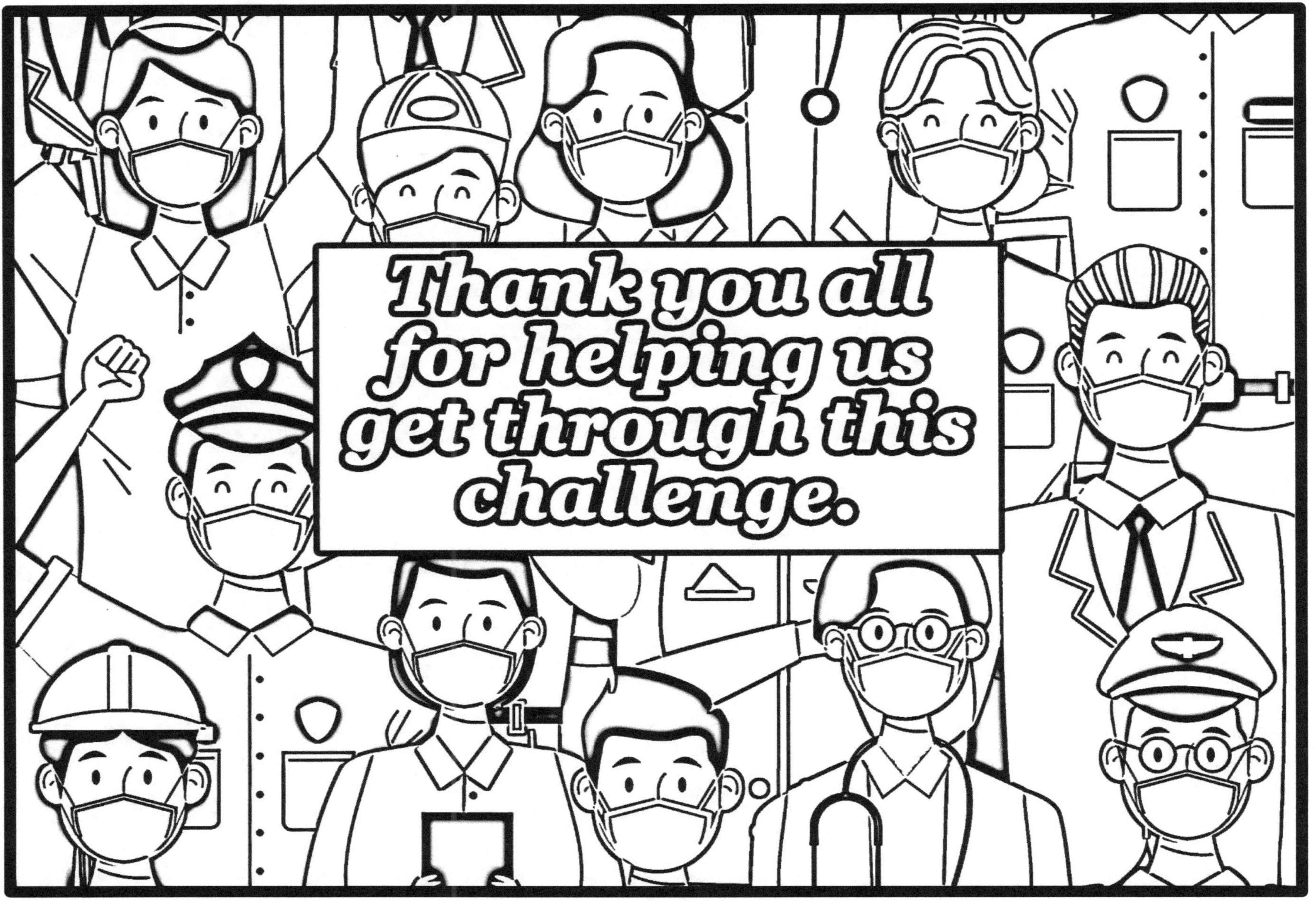

Thank you all
for helping us
get through this
challenge.

Artist Name:_______________________

Date:_______________________

Title:_______________________

Dedicated to:_______________________

Dear Artist,

Hope you had fun coloring these pages. Please send me an email and let me know what you thought or, if you would do me the very great favor, and write a review online where you got this coloring book.

Let me know if you have any ideas for additional illustrations or different coloring book themes.

I look forward to hearing from you.

All the best,

Rik Feeney
usabookcoach@gmail.com